To
HOMEOPATHY

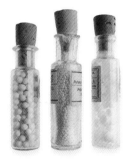

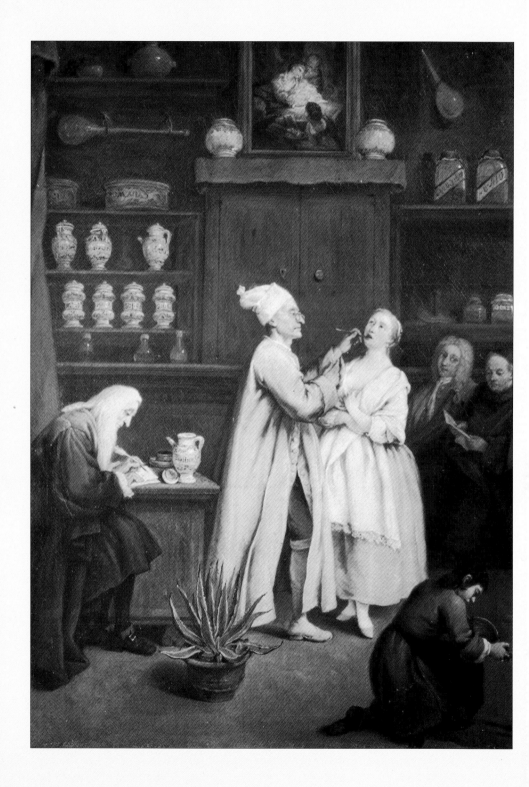

ILLUSTRATED ELEMENTS OF
HOMEOPATHY

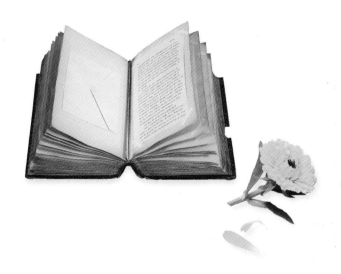

ILANA DANNHEISSER
AND PENNY EDWARDS

ELEMENT

First published in Great Britain in 1998 by
ELEMENT BOOKS LIMITED

This edition published 2002 by Element
An Imprint of HarperCollins*Publishers*
77–85 Fulham Palace Road
Hammersmith, London W6 8JB

Element™ is a trademark of HarperCollins*Publishers*

2 4 6 8 10 9 7 5 3 1

NOTE FROM THE PUBLISHER
*Any information given in this book is not intended to be taken
as a replacement for medical advice. Any person with a condition
requiring medical attention should consult a qualified
practitioner or therapist.*

Designed and created with
The Bridgewater Book Company Limited

Printed in Hong Kong by
Printing Express

British Library Cataloguing in Publication
data available

Library of Congress Cataloging-in-Publication data available

ISBN 0-00-713601-3

Acknowledgments

*The publisher would like to thank
the following for the use of pictures:*
A–Z Botanical Collection: 48c, 72r, 100c.
Bridgeman Art Library: 14b (British Library, London);
45bl (Musée D'Unterlinden, Colmar, France).
Bruce Coleman: 18r, 88b (Michael Fogden).
e.t. archive: 2, 10bl, 70b, 119.
Garden Picture Library: 16tr, 44c (Vaughan Fleming);
30c (Roger Hyam); 69l (Emma Peios); 104tr (Sunniva Harte);
105r (David Russell); 108c (Kim Blaxland); 122r (John Glover).
Hahnemann House Trust: 3, 10tl & br, 11bl & br.
Harry Smith Collection: 33b, 68l, 90r.
Image Bank: 75b.
Natural History Museum: 58tr, 82c, 106c.
NHPA: 54c, 92c.
Robert Harding Picture Library: 95t.
Science Photo Library: 102b.
Sue Cunningham Photographic: 64br, 84r.
Zefa UK/Stock Market: 6l, 16bl, 23b, 24bl & br, 39b, 40b, 41tl, 46b,
48bl, 59, 63tl, 64b, 67r, 71b, 74c, 80bl, 89t, 90bl, 93b, 98b, 109b.

Special thanks to
Rukshana Chenoy, Jessie Fuller, Simon Holden
Helen Jordan, Pat Knight, Julia Knight
Kay MacMullen, Andrew Milne, Sam Sains,
Steven Sparchett, Bob Sullivan, Jenny Sullivan,
Amelia Whitelaw, Ian Whitelaw
for help with photography

Authors' acknowledgments
To John Morgan and staff at Helios Pharmacy, Tunbridge Wells,
Kent, for all their help and support.

FRONTISPIECE
The Apothecary's Shop by Pietro Longhi

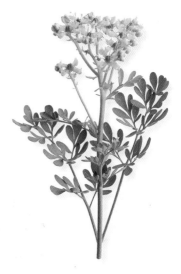

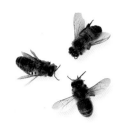

Contents

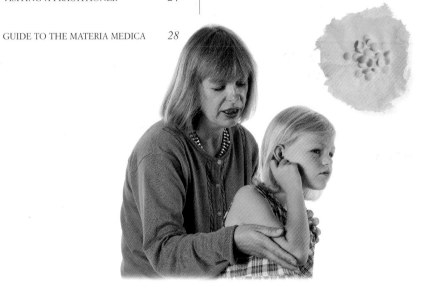

Introduction

AT THE PRESENT *time we see the flowering of a new way of thinking about our health and our lives. We have become more aware of the stresses we live with and what makes us ill, and many of us want to take a greater and more active role in our own health care. We are drawn to alternative or complementary methods of treatment because we want both to avoid the use of powerful drugs and to improve the quality of our health in order to prevent illness and disease.*

ABOVE *St. John's wort is one of many healing herbs.*

Although conventional medicine removes the symptoms of many common ailments and chronic diseases, it does not change the reason for our becoming ill in the first place, so we are likely to fall ill again. Homeopathy treats you, the individual, taking into account your inner nature, the causes of your illness, and the kind of stress you experience. While it cannot change the stressful world in which we live, it can help us to function better within it.

BELOW *Homeopathic remedies come in different forms, such as pills and powders.*

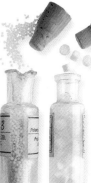

You will soon become familiar with the remedies and how to use them for different ailments. Each remedy covers a range of complaints, and there can be

ABOVE *The whole family may benefit from homeopathic remedies.*

more than one remedy for each ailment, so you will need to know how to look up the symptoms you wish to treat, and how to differentiate between the various remedies featured in this book. Learning how to use homeopathy does require some effort, but the results can be exciting and rewarding as you observe how quickly the body can heal itself.

How to Use This Book

This book is designed to help you treat many common minor ailments and injuries using homeopathy. Do not try to treat serious injuries or illnesses, recurrent infections, or deep-seated problems, which require the skills of a professional homeopath or other practitioner. Before using homeopathy, you need to be familiar with the basic principles of prescribing, and how to find the appropriate remedy. These subjects are covered in the first part of the book. The Materia Medica describes the remedies, followed by the Repertory Index of symptoms.

BELOW **The remedies that are used in homeopathic treatment are fully described in the Materia Medica, the main section of the book** (see p. 28).

In Materia Medica, remedies are listed in alphabetical order.

Your choice of remedy will depend on the individual person's "symptom picture" (see p. 15).

BELOW **The first part of the book acquaints the reader with the basic tenets of homeopathy and the ways in which remedies are prescribed and prepared.**

Homeopathy distinguishes between several different categories of symptoms.

The featured remedy is compared with other remedies that have similar properties.

Comprehensive listings make it possible to pinpoint the appropriate remedy in each case.

The source of the remedy is featured in full color.

RIGHT **The Repertory Index enables you to look up a particular symptom, or affected body part and find the appropriate remedy** (see p. 124).

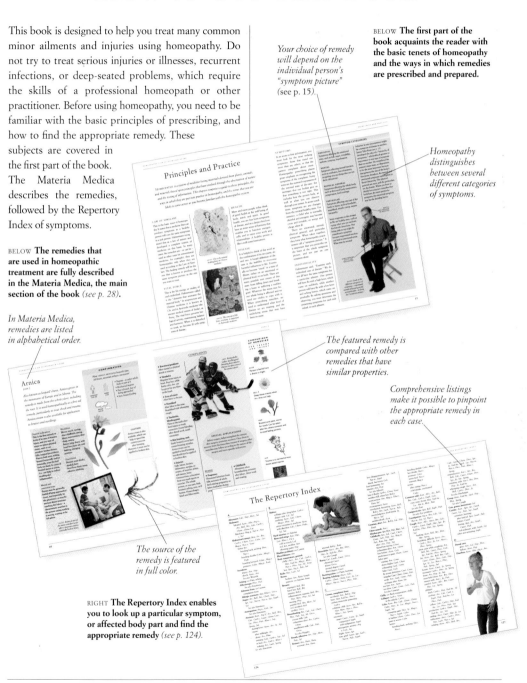

7

What Is Homeopathy?

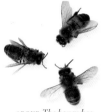

HOMEOPATHY *is a gentle yet effective form of treatment for many conditions, illnesses, and diseases. It is holistic in nature, which means that in determining treatment the whole person is considered as well as the specific problem or illness. The medicines, or remedies, used in homeopathy are minute doses of natural substances, which have been taken from plants, animals, or minerals.*

The word homeopathy comes from the Greek *homoios* meaning similar, and *patheia* meaning suffering, which together mean "similar suffering." So, in other words, homeopathy is the treatment of disease with substances that would, in a healthy person, elicit the symptoms of that disease. Conventional medicine is based on the opposite principle in that it combats a disease with strong doses of a medicine that will produce the opposite condition.

If we think of health as a state of ease, both mentally and physically, then illness is a state of "disease." Homeopathy works with the idea that we all have an innate ability to overcome "dis-ease." The energy, or vitality, that we all have within us enables us to grow, repair damaged tissue, respond to stresses in our environment, and generally function with a sense of well-being. When something happens to us that causes us to feel undue stress, we start to produce

symptoms: these are the expression of our "disease." By giving the appropriate homeopathic remedy, this natural healing energy is stimulated and the body can once again restore itself to balance and free itself of the symptoms that limited its normal or true function.

Homeopathic remedies allow the body to heal itself, without any of the harmful effects that can come from the use of conventional drugs. It also has a long-term benefit in that you raise your level of health generally, thus making you less susceptible to diseases in the future.

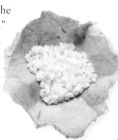

ABOVE *Many minerals, including potassium bichromate, are used to make homeopathic remedies.*

You can use this book to learn how to treat simple cases of accident and minor injury, and other ailments that are not complicated or life threatening. You should consult a professional homeopath if:
• Self-prescribing is not working, or your ailments are recurring.
• You are suffering from general stress and your resistance to infection is lowered.
• You have a range of complaints.
• You feel that your physical and emotional health is out of balance.
• You have a serious health problem. There are three basic levels of disease to consider.

RIGHT *The Indian cockle plant is used to make a tincture.*

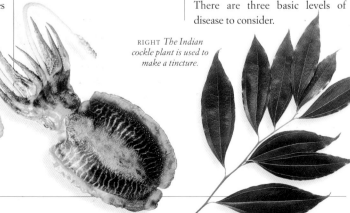

RIGHT *The cuttlefish is just one sea animal used in homeopathy.*

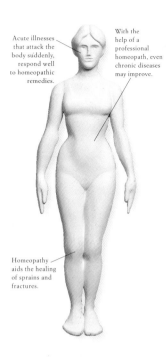

Acute illnesses that attack the body suddenly, respond well to homeopathic remedies.

With the help of a professional homeopath, even chronic diseases may improve.

Homeopathy aids the healing of sprains and fractures.

ABOVE *You can learn how to treat minor injuries from this book.*

ACCIDENTS AND INJURIES

When a complaint is the result of an external event, causing localized damage to tissues, you feel well, but temporarily indisposed. Homeopathy promotes rapid healing and restores vitality.
Examples: *Burns, bruises, cuts and grazes, insect stings, puncture wounds, sprains, strains, fractures, ill effects after dentistry or surgery.*

ACUTE ILLNESS

You feel generally healthy, have no major problems, but occasionally suffer from a cold or influenza. An acute illness comes on quickly, and usually goes away sooner or later by

itself. It could be a cold or minor infection, or a temporary imbalance caused by overexertion, travel, or overeating. The symptoms of infections and colds, such as fever, catarrh, and cough, are the natural response of the body's immune system. When treated homeopathically, the body works with, rather than suppresses, these symptoms. This in turn helps the body to recover health more quickly.
Examples: *Bacterial and viral infections, such as colds, coughs, bronchitis, tonsilitis, cystitis, ear infections, influenza, childhood diseases, and ailments from other causes such as exhaustion, sunstroke, travel sickness, hangover, nervousness prior to taking examinations.*

CHRONIC DISEASES

With chronic diseases, there is usually a history of suffering different complaints, one or more deep underlying causes, lowered vitality, and complaints that frequently recur (such as those acute illnesses mentioned above), or steadily get worse. There may be a medical diagnosis, but in many cases the person simply feels unwell, even though conventional tests detect nothing amiss. Homeopathy can treat deeper ongoing problems that have psychological and/or physical symptoms. These extreme conditions are more complex and require constitutional treatment from a professional qualified homeopath. The treatment can take several months, or years, depending on severity and how long the patient has been suffering.

Examples: *P.M.S. and other menstrual or hormonal disorders, infectious mononucleosis, rheumatism and arthritis, depression, debilitating or auto-immune diseases, as well as hyperactivity, behavioral problems, and learning difficulties in children.*

CAUTION

Always assess the seriousness of the ailment or injury. You must never substitute homeopathy for necessary medical attention, but you can give remedies while waiting for the doctor or ambulance to come. Serious infections, such as meningitis and pneumonia, can also be treated with homeopathy, but it is best to consult a professional homeopath as well as seeking immediate medical attention.

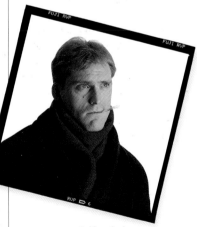

ABOVE *Colds and other acute illnesses respond well to homeopathy.*

Origins of Homeopathy

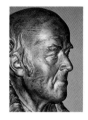

ABOVE *Samuel Hahnemann (1755–1843), the founder of homeopathy.*

THE PRACTICE OF present-day homeopathy is based on the work of Samuel Hahnemann, who first published his new theories 200 years ago. However, the natural principles underlying homeopathic thinking were identified as far back as Hippocrates, in the 5th century B.C.E., and were used by the ancient Egyptians. Indeed, the ancient medical systems of the East, such as Ayurvedic and Chinese medicine, bear some resemblance to homeopathy, in their view of treating the whole person and the idea of "vital force."

Samuel Hahnemann (1755–1843) was born in Meissen, in Saxony, and became a physician in 1779. At that time, the popular methods of orthodox treatment included bloodletting, purgation, emesis, and the use of large doses of chemical agents such as mercury and arsenic. Hahnemann soon realized that these methods were harmful and far from curative. Disillusioned, he stopped practicing medicine and became an open critic of these methods. To earn a living, he became a translator.

It was while translating William Cullen's *Materia Medica* that he read how quinine – derived from Peruvian Bark – was used to cure malaria because it was bitter. Hahnemann considered that other substances were bitter, but they did not cure malaria. He decided to test quinine on himself. As a result he began to get symptoms similar to those of malaria – such as intermittent fever – though not malaria itself. When he stopped taking quinine, his symptoms disappeared. This was the first "proving."

Hahnemann also knew that Hippocrates, who had lived nearly 2,000 years earlier, had stated that there were two methods of treating disease: by "similars" and by "opposites." This meant that you could give a medicine that would produce the opposite condition to the disease, or you could give a medicine that would produce the same symptoms as the disease. Through his own proving, Hahnemann realized the connection: a medicine capable of producing symptoms in a healthy person will cure similar symptoms in a diseased person. He called this principle the "Law of Similars," derived from the Latin *Similia similibus curentur*, meaning "Let like be cured by like."

Hahnemann began to test other substances on his family, friends, and students. They rigorously and systematically noted all the symptoms that occurred after taking the medicine, being equally careful to eliminate any symptoms that were already present. This was how the action of remedies was discovered.

Since many of the substances Hahnemann used were poisonous in their natural form (mercury, for example), he began diluting them

C.470–400 B.C.E.	1493–1542	1755–1843	1800–1880
HIPPOCRATES *Greece.* Father of medicine; conceives of two methods of healing – by contraries and by similars.	**PARACELSUS** *Switzerland.* Born Theophrastus Bombastus von Hohenheim. Biochemist, physiologist, pathologist; introduces essential ideas upon which modern medicine is based; anticipates the fundamental principles of homeopathy.	**SAMUEL HAHNEMANN** *Germany.* Founds and develops present-day homeopathic practice.	**CONSTANTINE HERING** *U.S.A.* Develops "Law of Cure" and writes *Hering's Guiding Symptoms.*

to reduce their toxic effects. At a certain point, they were no longer poisonous, but they seemed also to lose their curative action. As a result of further experimentation, he introduced a new step into the procedure: at each stage of dilution, he began to succuss – or repeatedly strike – the containers against a hard, elastic surface. Hahnemann found that this process not only took away the noxious effects of certain medicines but also enabled them to heal more effectively. In conjunction with dilution negating the poisonous effects of a substance, succussion transfers the energy pattern of the substance to the liquid, so you do not need to take a material dose. Hahnemann called this process of dilution and succussion "dynamization."

He frequently wrote about his discoveries, but was ridiculed by the powerful establishment of his day. Nevertheless, he had many satisfied and enthusiastic patients. Over the years, Hahnemann wrote a definitive work about the principles and practices of homeopathic treatment entitled *The Organon of the Healing Art*. The sixth, and last, edition of this important and groundbreaking work is still much used by contemporary homeopaths.

MAJOR FIGURES

FREDERICK QUIN
1799–1879, Britain
Studied with Hahnemann and brought homeopathy to Britain; established the British Homeopathic Society; founded the London Homeopathic Hospital (1849).

CONSTANTINE HERING
1800–1880, U.S.A.
Trained in orthodox medicine, but adopted homeopathy; proved many new remedies; brought homeopathy to the United States where he helped to set up the Hahnemann Medical College; wrote *Hering's Guiding Symptoms*, in ten volumes.

DR. JAMES TYLER KENT
1849–1916, U.S.A.
Practiced orthodox medicine until he discovered and adopted homeopathy; developed the *Repertory of Symptoms* (1877) in which all symptoms are listed systematically with the remedies that produce those symptoms, and it is still used as a major reference work and tool by today's homeopaths; introduced higher potencies; developed the idea of constitutional prescribing.

DR. JAMES COMPTON BURNETT
1849–1900, Britain
Received medical degrees in Vienna (1869) and Glasgow (1872), and excelled in the study and application of anatomy. Converted to homeopathy after much doubt and skepticism; developed and expanded homeopathic therapeutics; introduced new remedies, the use of organopathy (the practice of using homeopathic medicines in the treatment of pathological conditions of specific organs of the body) and nosodes (remedies made from human tissue taken from individuals with specific diseases), and treatment of ill effects of vaccination.

TIMOTHY F. ALLEN
19th century, U.S.A.
Gathered all information from provings and accidental poisonings into a comprehensive *Encyclopedia of Materia Medica* (1874).

DR. JOHN C. CLARKE
1853–1932, U.S.A.
Wrote *A Dictionary of Practical Materia Medica* (1900), listing all known remedies.

DR. EDWARD BACH
1886–1936, Britain
Bacteriologist and homeopath; created the Bach Flower Essence remedies.

1799–1879	1849–1916	1849–1900	1886–1936
 FREDERICK QUIN *Britain.* Brings homeopathy to Britain.	JAMES TYLER KENT *U.S.A.* Develops Kent's Repertory (*Repertory of Symptoms*).	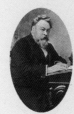 DR. JAMES COMPTON BURNETT *Britain.* Synthesizes different approaches.	DR. EDWARD BACH *Britain.* Creates Bach Flower Essence remedies.

Homeopathy around the World

ABOVE *Global travel has led to an increased awareness of homeopathic medicine.*

THE RECENT *expansion of homeopathy around the globe has occurred largely in the last 20–30 years. With a growing awareness of ecological concerns and a desire for a way of life that is good for both body and mind has come the trend toward natural and holistic medicine. Travel around the world has become, for many, routine, and therefore these ideas are taking hold in different countries at an ever-increasing rate. Here we discuss the current status of homeopathy in various parts of the world.*

AUSTRALIA AND NEW ZEALAND

Homeopathy is well established and spreading quickly, with a mandate given to professional homeopathic societies by the government to develop courses with approval for federal funding.

CANADA

The Canadian Medical Association has a "Complementary Medicine Section," that includes homeopathy. Homeopathic medicines are widely available in pharmacies.

CZECH REPUBLIC

Homeopathy was accepted within the conventional medical society in this country in 1990.

FRANCE

An estimated 36 percent of the population uses homeopathy. It is taught in some medical schools, as well as dental, veterinary, midwifery schools, and schools of pharmacy.

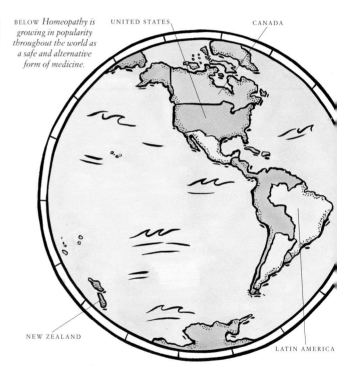

BELOW *Homeopathy is growing in popularity throughout the world as a safe and alternative form of medicine.*

UNITED STATES

CANADA

NEW ZEALAND

LATIN AMERICA

GREAT BRITAIN

There are 5 homeopathic hospitals in Great Britain, more than 500 registered members of the Society of Homeopaths, and hundreds more licensed practitioners. Homeopathic medicines have been recognized and used by the royal family since the 19th century. A large percentage of general practitioners are interested in receiving some training in, or referring their patients to, complementary therapies.

GREECE

There is a clinic and training school set up by George Vithoulkas, who is commonly recognized as one of the most important contributors to modern homeopathy. His writings and teachings have greatly influenced many well-known and international teachers and practitioners of homeopathy.

NETHERLANDS

Homeopathy is gaining in popularity with medical doctors, and the standard of practice is high.

HUNGARY

In 1994, the Hungarian Homeopathic Medical Association had more than 300 members.

ISRAEL

Homeopathy is practiced in many small clinics and some of their larger hospitals.

UNITED STATES

Interest in homeopathy is mushrooming. Between 1,000 and 2,000 medical doctors practice homeopathy, and there are about 1,000 naturopathic physicians, as well as veterinarians, dentists, and chiropractors who use homeopathy. There are at least 15 training institutions, 9 manufacturers of homeopathic medicines, 6 homeopathic organizations, and 5 examining/certifying boards across the country.

GERMANY

Ten percent of doctors specialize in homeopathy. There are 3,000 natural health practitioners who specialize in homeopathy, and approximately 98 percent of pharmacies sell homeopathic medicines (largely the result of the development of homeopathy in Western Germany before unification).

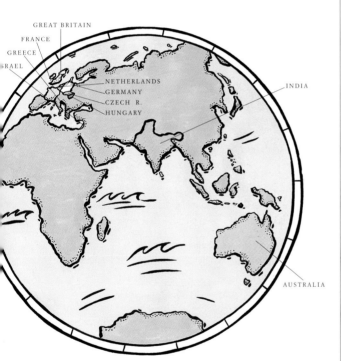

INDIA

Homeopathy is recognized as a separate branch of medicine. There are about 300,000 fulltime homeopaths, over 100,000 doctor homeopaths, and over 120 colleges providing homeopathic training.

WORLDWIDE INTEREST

Interest in homeopathy is developing in the Scandinavian countries, Poland, Russia, Japan, and South Africa.

LATIN AMERICA

There are many thousands of homeopaths in Latin America, especially in Mexico, Argentina, and Brazil, and the standards of practice are high. In Mexico there are two homeopathic medical schools, one with more than 800 students. Homeopathic medicines are available in many pharmacies.

Principles and Practice

HOMEOPATHY *is a system of medicine (using materials derived from plants, animals, and minerals) based upon principles that have evolved through the observation of nature and the testing of information. This chapter comprises a guide to these principles, the ways in which they are put into practice in homeopathy, and the terms that you are likely to come across as you become familiar with the homeopathic system.*

LAW OF SIMILARS

This is the basic tenet of homeopathy. It states that a medicine that can produce symptoms in a healthy person will cure the same symptoms in a sick person. Hahnemann recognized this as a law of nature and developed a complete system of medicine on this basis. In many cases, the remedies are – or can be – used in other ways (in conventional medicine, for example); they are homeopathic only when they are used according to the Law of Similars. The healing remedy will be the one that is known to produce the same symptom picture as the one you want to treat.

VITAL FORCE

This is the life energy, or vitality, of each individual. Hahnemann called it the "dynamis that animates the material body." In acupuncture and Chinese medicine it is known as *Chi*, and in Ayurvedic medicine (the ancient medical system of India), as *Prana*. The vital force governs biological activity, maintaining balance and harmony. When it is disturbed or weak, we become ill with symptoms of disease.

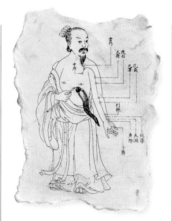

ABOVE *Chi is the natural healing force in Chinese medicine.*

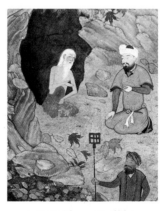

ABOVE *The concept of life force, or prana, is important in Ayurvedic medicine.*

HEALTH

More and more people today think of good health as the well-being of body, mind, and spirit. In good health, you are free from symptoms of disease, and on a deeper level you have an inner sense of harmony that enables you to function energetically, and to enjoy your work and relationships. A healthy person is like a well-tuned instrument.

DISEASE

It is helpful to think of this word as the combination of its two parts, *dis* and *ease*. A broad definition of disease is the inability to overcome harmful influences in life. Eventually we become "stuck" in a state of illness, either on an emotional or physical level, or on both. There are many possible root causes of this state, from falling down and breaking a bone to suffering a sudden grief. Whatever the stress may be, our whole being is affected and we need our vitality to cope with it. When prescribing remedies, we need to understand what level of disease we are treating, and the underlying stress that may have been its cause.

SYMPTOMS

In an acute or first aid situation, you must look for the most striking symptoms, those that stand out more than any others, or that the patient complains about most. Homeopathic prescribing places great emphasis on recognizing the symptoms of the complaint. Symptoms are the outward expressions of the internal state of dis-ease: the messages that our bodies give us that something is not right. This includes how the person feels, as well as what you can observe through your senses. In acute conditions, symptoms are any changes from the normal healthy state. For instance, a child who is normally cheerful and energetic may become cross and irritable, or weepy and clingy, when ill.

There are emotional, mental, physical general, and particular symptoms. When taken together, they form what homeopathic practitioners call a "symptom picture." It is important that you prescribe on the basis of the whole symptom picture, and not just on one symptom alone.

INDIVIDUALITY

Hahnemann said, "Examine each individual case of disease." We do not all have the same symptoms for a particular ailment. One person will have flu with a high fever, which came on suddenly, while another person will have flu with a low fever and aching bones, which came on gradually. By asking questions and observing, you must determine the presenting symptoms for each individual, in each ailment.

SYMPTOM CATEGORIES

EMOTIONAL
Symptoms affecting the emotional state, such as fear, anger, irritability, sadness, weeping, hopelessness.

MENTAL
Symptoms affecting mental function, such as confusion, loss of memory, imagining you see things that are not there (delusions).

PHYSICAL GENERAL
Symptoms affecting the whole body, such as abnormal body temperature, perspiration, food cravings.

PARTICULAR
Symptoms affecting one part of the body or tissue, such as headache, nosebleed, muscle cramp, nausea (stomach).

Some responses to the stresses in life are healthy ones, such as crying when you are sad from the loss of a loved one. Not being able to cry might be considered a symptom because suppressed emotion can lead to emotional stress. What may be normal

behavior in one circumstance might be a symptom of disease in another. James Tyler Kent (*see p. 11*) developed the idea of a "hierarchy of symptoms," which affords greater or importance to one type of symptom than to another. He considered the person's inner state, or disposition, to be the most important because that governs the rest of the body's functions; therefore, the mental and emotional symptoms rank highest in Kent's hierarchy. The physical generals are next, and the particulars are the lowest. When you have to decide between two remedies that both have the same particular symptom, the emotional symptom may be the deciding factor.

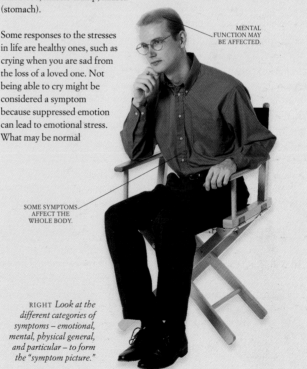

MENTAL FUNCTION MAY BE AFFECTED.

SOME SYMPTOMS AFFECT THE WHOLE BODY.

RIGHT *Look at the different categories of symptoms – emotional, mental, physical general, and particular – to form the "symptom picture."*

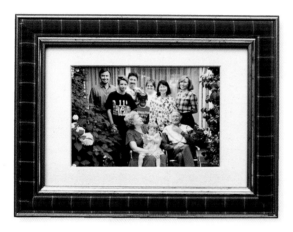

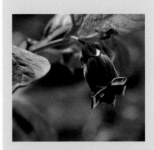

ABOVE *Deadly nightshade was one of the first provings by Hahnemann.*

SUSCEPTIBILITY

We all respond to different influences in different ways at different times. When our energy is low, we are more likely to get an infection. We all have individual areas of weakness. Such a weakness might be a tendency to suffer from ear infections, digestive upsets, or swollen glands. If we are susceptible, or sensitive, to a particular trigger, it can affect us on any level of our health; the trigger might be anything from cold weather to a

BELOW *Work pressures may cause disease to manifest itself in certain individuals.*

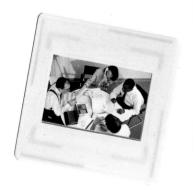

ABOVE *A homeopath will inquire into a person's family history before prescribing a remedy.*

demanding boss, and can lead to stress or disease. Recurrent problems may indicate a constitutional susceptibility, or weakness, which must be treated by a professional, qualified homeopath.

CONSTITUTION

Hahnemann recognized that chronic diseases originate from a person's constitution, which is the person's individual physical, emotional, and intellectual makeup. The constitution is determined by both the genes a person inherits and environmental influences. When prescribing constitutionally, the homeopath looks deeper into the person's history to find the pattern of reactions typical for that individual. Treating on this profound level helps to prevent the development of diseases, correct any imbalances that may exist, and maintain good health and a strong immune system.

A "proving" is the term used to describe the testing of the action of a remedy on healthy people (we do not test on animals), so that its curative properties can also be known. Hahnemann refined this method into carefully controlled experiments and formulated strict guidelines for its procedure; these are written in *The Organon of Healing Art* (*see p. 11*). Many of the first provings tested substances that were already known to have medicinal effects, such as the plant *Belladonna* (deadly nightshade). Hahnemann's followers carried out many more provings, so the range of possible remedies continued to expand. At present within the professional homeopathic community there is a great interest in developing new remedies from previously untested substances. Among the newer remedies that have been proved according to Hahnemann's guidelines, are hydrogen from the periodic table, scorpion from the animal kingdom, and the plant *Brassica* (rape seed).

THE MINIMUM DOSE

This is the basic rule governing how much of the remedy to give. That is, you give only enough of any particular remedy to initiate a curative response from the patient. This varies according to the level of disease and the severity of the complaint. Full instructions about this can be found in the section on dosage (*see p. 22*). This is extremely important, because if you take too much of a remedy, you may start to develop new symptoms (a proving) and counteract the good work of the remedy!

THE SINGLE REMEDY

In classical homeopathic prescribing it is usual to give only one remedy at a time, though it can be repeated. By giving only one dose at a time, you can easily see if there is improvement. If there is no curative response, or if the symptom picture alters, you may need to move on to a different remedy.

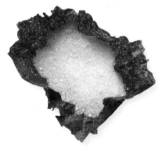

ABOVE *Take only one remedy at a time so that you are able to see more easily if there is an improvement.*

RIGHT *Any remedy should be carefully measured because taking too much may cause new symptoms to develop.*

THE MATERIA MEDICA

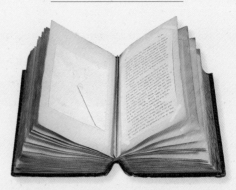

The *Materia Medica* books contain the information about remedies. The name means medical matter or material. All the information comes from provings, and it is arranged according to the order of symptoms: mental/emotional, physical general, and particulars of the body from the head downward. There are many versions of *Materia Medica*, written by homeopaths who give their own clinical verification of the therapeutic

ABOVE *Books of* Materia Medica *have provided comprehensive remedies for hundreds of years.*

action of the remedies. When you find there are a few remedies indicated for the complaint you wish to treat, you refer to the *Materia Medica* for the complete picture of each remedy. You can then select the one that best fits the overall picture of your complaint.

THE REPERTORY

A repertory is an index of symptoms, and it constitutes the basic tool of homeopathy. From provings, we see that different symptoms are produced by different substances. Dr. James Tyler Kent (*see p. 11*) arranged all this information to make it easy for those suffering from a particular ailment to look up a symptom and to see which remedies would be able to produce that symptom and therefore help to cure it.

The Repertory also shows you remedies whose ability to cure a particular symptom has been clinically verified.

Kent's Repertory is systematically arranged according to his hierarchy of symptoms (*see p. 11*). This is the repertory that is most widely used among today's homeopaths, though there are other versions that may also be consulted.

Preparing and Finding a Remedy

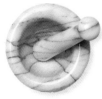

THE MEDICINES *used in homeopathy are made from the three kingdoms of the natural world – plant, animal, and mineral. Many of the substances used are known to have powerful effects, and when taken in large material doses are poisonous. Examples of these are the deadly nightshade plant, the minerals arsenic and mercury, and venom from poisonous snakes and spiders.*

ABOVE *Insoluble source material is ground up with lactose to make the tincture.*

There are generally two ways of preparing the remedies, the first for plants, the second for minerals and other nonplant substances. Plants are macerated and soaked in a mixture of alcohol and water, which becomes the "mother tincture."

Thereafter, the mixture is diluted by adding one drop of the tincture to 99 drops of alcohol and water; it is then succussed. This is called a 1c potency: the c stands for centesimal because the substance is diluted one part in one hundred. The process is repeated by taking one drop of the 1c mixture, diluting it with 99 drops of alcohol and water, and succussing it. This is the 2c potency. Each progressive dilution and succussion yields the next higher potency. Nonplant substances are diluted initially by trituration (grinding up) with lactose, or milk sugar. Still at the ratio of one part in one hundred, this procedure is repeated up to 3c, at which stage the lactose/mineral mixture can be dissolved. Ensuing steps are then carried out in the same manner as for liquid potencies.

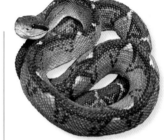

ABOVE *Poisonous snakes, such as this bushmaster, are the source of some remedies.*

If a substance is diluted by one part in ten, it is called a decimal potency and the letter x is used to denote this, i.e. 6x, 12x, etc.

REMEDY DILUTION AND POTENTIZATION

Any substance used to make a homeopathic remedy must be diluted in a solution and succussed. This process is called potentization. The more a solution is potentized, the more powerful it becomes.

The mother tincture is prepared from the source material.

One drop of the tincture is diluted with 99 drops of alcohol and water.

The remedy is then succussed. This makes the 1c potency.

Using the 1c potency, the process is then repeated to reach the required potency.

The potentized remedies are made into pills, powders, creams, or ointments.

DYNAMIZATION

In order to reduce the toxic effects of substances without losing their curative value, homeopaths use a process called dynamization – a method of dilution developed by Hahnemann. Through his experiments, Hahnemann found that not only did dynamization have the required result of negating the toxic effect of poisons, but in some way it enhanced their remedial effects. By experimenting further, he found that other substances, which in their natural form are completely inert (such as salt, silica, and *Lycopodium*), also yielded curative effects when subjected to this process.

The effects of dynamization reflect a present-day law of chemistry – the Arndt-Schultz Law (also known as hormesis) – which decrees that strong doses of a substance can kill, medium doses inhibit (these are the doses used by modern medicine), and small doses stimulate (the homeopathic application). For example, very weak concentrations of iodine, bromine, mercuric chloride, and arsenious acid will stimulate yeast growth, medium doses of these substances will inhibit yeast growth, and large doses will kill the yeast.

LEFT Aconite *may prove to be the correct remedy for a person with fever caused by a cold wind.*

FINDING A REMEDY

As we have seen, the basic principle of homeopathy is that a medicine that can produce symptoms of disease in a healthy person will cure the same symptoms in someone who is ill. Each remedy used in homeopathy is known for its own kind of action – the symptoms it creates; this is known as the remedy's "symptom picture." When treating a patient, you must first know the symptoms of the illness, and then find the remedy that can produce the most similar symptoms. When you have matched, as nearly as possible, the symptom picture of the remedy to the symptom picture of the illness, you will have found a well-indicated homeopathic remedy.

Finding the curative remedy is somewhat like detective work. First you need to observe the changes in

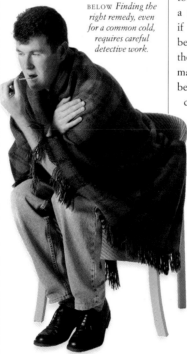

BELOW *Finding the right remedy, even for a common cold, requires careful detective work.*

the patient's behavior and feelings. Use your own senses: what do you see, hear, smell, touch, feel? For example, is there a sudden high fever with red face and cold hands, barking cough, anxious facial expression? You then find out how the person feels: hot, with a bursting headache and burning sore throat, and dry, with a thirst for cold drinks. The person says "I am going to die," though you know it is just a cold. You then try to find out if there is a direct relationship between an event and the onset of these symptoms. For example, you may discover that a few hours before, this person became very cold while walking in the cold, dry air, or experienced a shock or fright. All of this information is used together to form your symptom picture.

You then find out which remedy covers the symptoms: rapid onset of fever, burning heat, dry sore throat, barking cough, desire for cold drinks, fear of death. You find that the remedy *Aconite* covers all these symptoms, and that a frequent cause of the symptoms is being in a cold wind. Given in the correct dose, *Aconite* will therefore promote rapid recovery.

Prescribing a Remedy

A good result in homeopathy depends on the prescriber's ability to match the symptoms
of the disease with those of a remedy. This requires being familiar with symptoms as
well as remedies. Sometimes a person's symptoms are subtle, and we can miss an
important indication because we do not recognize it as part of the symptom picture.

Here is a step-by-step guide to basic self-prescribing, to help you find the best-indicated remedy for your complaint.

1 NOTING THE SYMPTOMS

The key to successful prescribing lies in your ability to recognize the important symptoms of the illness, which distinguish one remedy picture from another. When suffering from a complaint, everyone will experience different changes in the way they usually feel. Sometimes the symptoms are very clearly recognizable, but at other times you have to use your powers of observation. If you are prescribing for someone else, you need to know what to ask as well as what to observe.

- ONSET: How did it start? Slowly or suddenly?
- CAUSATIVE FACTORS: Was there a trigger, physical or emotional? For example, becoming chilled or experiencing a strong emotion.
- EMOTIONS: What is your mood? Has it changed from how it usually is? For example, a child who is normally independent craves attention.
- LOCATION: Where are you affected? Head, nose, throat, ear, chest, stomach, bowels?

FIVE ESSENTIAL STEPS

There are five essential steps in prescribing a remedy:

- Note the symptoms.
- Look up the symptoms.
- Decide which remedy is appropriate.
- Decide the dose, and how often and when to repeat it.
- Evaluate the result.

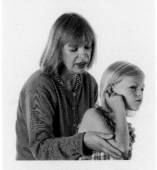

ABOVE *Some physical symptoms are clearly recognizable, such as earache.*

- SENSATIONS: What does it feel like? A tight band, bruised, on fire?
- PAIN: What kind of pain do you feel? Sharp, throbbing, sore? What do you do to make it feel better? Apply cold or heat, loosen clothing, bend double, apply pressure?

- MODALITIES: What makes you feel better or worse? Think about time of day, temperature, movement, position, pressure, touch, drafts, drinking, eating.
- COUGH: What kind of cough is it? Dry, hard, loose, painful? When is it better or worse? In open air, in a warm room, when swallowing hot or cold drinks?
- DISCHARGE: What is the color and odor? Is it bland or irritating? Yellow, green, clear?
- APPETITE: Do you want any particular food? Sweet, sour, spicy, salty?
- THIRST: Are you more, or less, thirsty than usual? Do you want to drink cold or hot drinks? How much? Any particular kind?
- TEMPERATURE: Do you feel hot or cold? Is the way you feel inside the same as the way the skin feels to the touch? Does it vary from one place to another? Hot face with cold hands and feet, for example.
- VISIBLE CHANGES: Are there other visible signs, such as redness, swelling, skin eruptions?
- OTHER SYMPTOMS: Are there two or more symptoms that happen at the same time, such as headache with cold sweat?
Which are the really strong, clear symptoms?

2 LOOKING UP THE SYMPTOMS

The name of a disease is just a convenient way of classifying a collection of symptoms.

Think about what the actual symptoms are, then refer to the Repertory Index *(see pp.126–133)*.

In order to use the Repertory Index, the symptom you have needs to be expressed in the way that it is listed. For instance, you have a high fever, but do not want to drink anything. This would be listed under Fever, thirst absent. The main symptom is fever, and "thirst absent" is a distinguishing characteristic. The best symptoms to use are the ones you feel most sure of.

The symptoms are listed alphabetically, either by complaint or by part of the body, e.g. boils, throat.

The Repertory is a general guide to the symptoms. The most important symptoms are there, and they will direct you to the most appropriate remedies for your complaint, but you must read the Materia Medica for the fullest description of the remedy, and to confirm your particular choice.

For each symptom write down all the remedies listed.

ONE AT A TIME

Be optimistic: If you give the chosen remedy and the person does not improve, you can always try one of the other remedies on your shortlist!
But remember – give only one remedy at a time.

3 DECIDING WHICH REMEDY TO USE

When you have written down all the remedies for each symptom, find the remedy that is for all or most of the symptoms. There may be more than one. If you have too many to choose from, it is most likely that your symptom choices were not precise enough. In this case, look again at the symptoms you have chosen and determine how strong they are. Choose again, using fewer but more specific symptoms. For instance, the symptom "Headache" is too general – it will give too many remedies to choose from. Try to find something characteristic about it, such as "Better for cold application." The more precise and sure the symptom, the more likely it is you will find a useful remedy.

At this stage your choice of remedy should be narrowed down to a shortlist of two or three. Then find the description of each remedy picture in the Materia Medica section. It is not important to have all the symptoms in the remedy picture, but it is important that most of them are there. The whole remedy picture is like a completed puzzle, and your complaint will

form only part of this picture: you do not have to have all the pieces of the puzzle, but the pieces you do have must fit. If after reading about the remedies on your shortlist you are satisfied that one of them is the most suitable remedy, your search is complete. If you are not, you have to go back and check your symptom list to see if you have missed something important. Reading about the remedies will help you to recognize what sorts of symptoms apply.

Sometimes you will have more than one good choice, and you will then have to differentiate between remedies. Examine them again, this time comparing them to each other more directly. Look at the section on comparison of remedies: this will give you an idea of the important indications of each remedy, and how to decide between them.

Potencies

In acute prescribing, it is best to use the lower potencies, 6c, 12c, 30c. If these potencies are working well but you need to repeat frequently, and you are sure of the remedy picture, you can use the 200c potency. Dosage guidelines are given in Step 4.

RIGHT *A "headache" is too general a symptom to look up in the Repertory Index. Be more specific about its symptoms.*

DOES NAUSEA ACCOMPANY HEADACHE?

DOES HOLDING THE HEAD MAKE IT FEEL BETTER?

DO YOU HAVE EYESTRAIN?

4 DECIDING THE DOSE

Remember that one of the main principles of prescribing homeopathically is the "minimum dose." This means giving only the amount required to initiate a healing response. This will depend on the seriousness and urgency of the complaint: the more serious and urgent, the more frequent the dose (*see also* Potencies in Step 3).

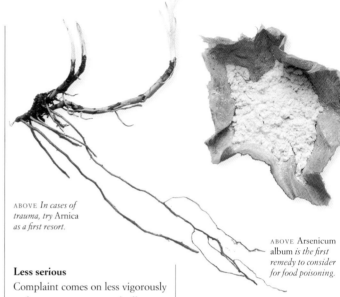

ABOVE *In cases of trauma, try* Arnica *as a first resort.*

ABOVE Arsenicum album *is the first remedy to consider for food poisoning.*

Very serious, urgent

There is a sudden, immediate, or intense onset, and it is usually accompanied by severe pain.

Give one dose every 5–30 minutes; stop on improvement; repeat as needed. Change the remedy if the picture changes.

• EXAMPLE *If you severely sprain or break your ankle in an accident, your body will respond immediately and vigorously with pain, bruising, and swelling.* Arnica *is the first remedy to think of for traumatic injury, so you take* Arnica *every 5–10 minutes until you begin to feel better. You will not have miraculously healed the ankle, but you will feel a distinct change once the immediate trauma subsides. You may need to give a different remedy later, depending on the symptoms* (see Injuries, p. 130).

Serious

The complaint comes on suddenly, but is less intense and painful. Give one dose every 1–2 hours.

• EXAMPLE *A case of food poisoning, with vomiting and diarrhea several hours after eating. The symptoms point to* Arsenicum, *which you give every 1–2 hours until symptoms abate.*

Less serious

Complaint comes on less vigorously and progresses more gradually. One dose every 4–8 hours, or 3–4 times per day.

• EXAMPLE *This is the pattern commonly seen in most colds, flu, childhood diseases, teething, and in the second phase of injury.*

Childbirth

Childbirth can progress slowly or quickly, but the process can be greatly helped by homeopathic remedies. Follow the basic rules below to decide how frequently to give the indicated remedy.

Basic rules for all situations

• Judge the urgency of the situation: the more intense, the more frequent the dose.

CAUTION

Always get medical attention when urgently needed.

• Increase the gap between doses when you notice some improvement in the condition.
• Stop altogether when there is definite improvement.
• Repeat as needed – if the person relapses and becomes worse again.

TIP

If you have given six doses without improvement, you probably need a different remedy.

Before and after surgery

The usual recommended dose is one dose of the remedy the night before, one the morning of the surgery, and one after, depending on the nature of the surgery. Refer to the Repertory and Materia Medica for the appropriate remedy, and further instructions on pre- and postoperative use of homeopathy.

5 EVALUATING THE RESULT

How do you know if the remedy has worked well or not? What can be considered a good reaction?

If you are prescribing for yourself, you will probably know if you begin to feel better or not. The pains or other symptoms will ease up, or you will feel lighter, your mood may lift, or you may fall asleep, which is a common reaction. Sleep is usually a healing process (an exception to this is if you are treating a head concussion). If you start to feel better "in yourself" even though the physical symptoms have not changed, the remedy is having a healing effect. The improvement of the emotional state is often noticeable before physical improvement. This demonstrates that healing works outwardly from within.

If you are treating someone else, you have to sharpen your powers of observation. How does the person seem to you? The person's change in mood is usually the first sign: more, or less, cheerful, anxious, distressed, relaxed, energetic, peaceful, and so forth. Other symptoms need to be asked about: Are the pains better? Is the fever lower? If you are treating a young child who cannot answer these questions, you must assess the child's mood and demeanor. Any sign that the person is more at ease indicates a good reaction to the remedy.

What if the remedy works well to begin with but, when you repeat as needed, it does not work again? There are two possibilities: if the symptom picture has changed, you may need a different remedy; if it has not, you may need to try a stronger potency of the same remedy. Look again and see if there is a change of symptoms.

THE DANGERS OF OVERPRESCRIBING

To use homeopathy effectively, it is important to follow the instructions for dosage very carefully. Homeopathy works on the principle of the minimum dose. That is, you take only the amount necessary to initiate the healing process. More is not necessarily better. If you take the remedy too often it can stop working. Read the basic principles of prescribing before you begin to prescribe.

BELOW *Once the remedy begins to work you may fall into a deep sleep.*

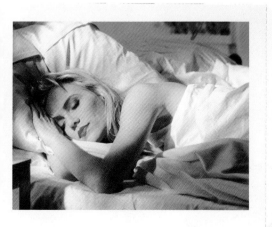

IS THE FEVER LOWER?

ARE YOU MORE RELAXED?

HAS THE PAIN LESSENED?

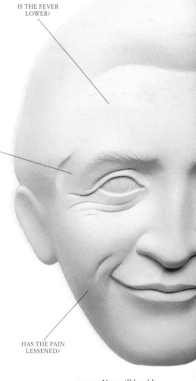

ABOVE *You will be able to recognize your mental mood lightening.*

Visiting a Practitioner

IF YOU DECIDE you would like to be treated by a professional homeopath, you will find the process of prescribing follows a similar pattern for your treatment to that used for acute self-prescribing. Here are some pointers about when to go and what to expect from your practitioner.

Do you have expectations of homeopathic treatment? Do you consider it to be a magic bullet? A miraculous cure? A lengthy and prolonged course of treatment? All of these are possible, but the truth is not as black and white. There is a range of factors that determines how quickly you will be "cured."

Homeopathic constitutional treatment is based on a person's total symptom picture. This includes present and past medical history, genetic makeup, and current symptoms – physical (general and particular), emotional, and mental.The first consultation can last from one to two hours, during which time the homeopath is learning about you and the pattern of your ill health. You may find that the homeopath's questions

WHEN TO CONSULT A PROFESSIONAL HOMEOPATH

- If you feel that your physical and emotional health is out of balance.
- After an acute illness, to balance your immune system.
- When self-prescribing is not working, or when minor ailments are recurrent.
- You are suffering from general stress and your resistance to infection is lowered.
- You have a range of complaints.
- You have a serious health problem.
- To maintain a good level of health.

are unusual, or seem to you to be irrelevant. The choice of remedy will be based on a detailed analysis of your individual emotional and physical reactions to a variety of stimuli in your environment, in both health and disease.

Some homeopaths may refer to a constitutional picture as a homeopathic "type." This means that the symptoms and reactions are understood as a recognized pattern of general physical, particular, and mental/emotional symptoms. For example, a *Calcarea carbonica* type is likely to be slightly overweight, fair-haired, fearful, and lacking in self-confidence, as well as perspire on the head while sleeping and have a strong desire for boiled eggs. The recognized pattern correlates with the picture of the remedy

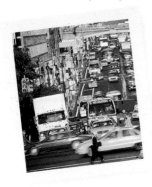

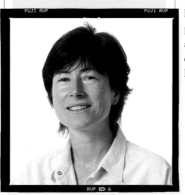

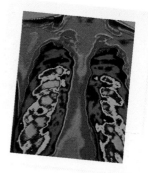

ABOVE, LEFT, AND RIGHT
A homeopath will look at your total symptom picture before prescribing treatment. This will include family history, lifestyle, and current health.

and is verified by clinical experience. Viewing a person as a "type" can be helpful in the objective understanding of the pattern; but because of the complexities involved in constitutional prescribing, the constitutional remedy may often be different from what is indicated merely by "type."

The remedies in this book can all be used as "acute" remedies, and many of them are commonly used in constitutional prescribing as well; you will get some idea of the "type" from the symptoms listed, especially the mental/emotional, physical generals, and modalities. When you consult your homeopath to be treated on the fundamental level of your constitutional susceptibility (*see* "Principles and Practice" section *on pp. 14–15*), the homeopath will recognize that the acute remedy you have selected for your illness will be in some way related to your constitutional picture.

However, since there are many subtleties and variations in people's natures it is important to see a professionally qualified homeopath, in order to be sure that the remedy selected is the most indicated one.

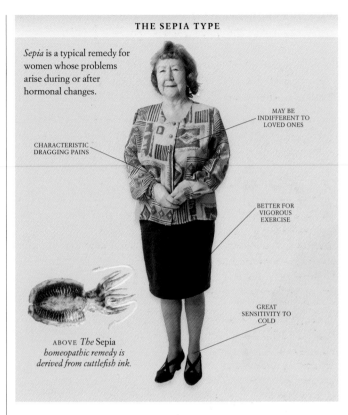

THE SEPIA TYPE

Sepia is a typical remedy for women whose problems arise during or after hormonal changes.

MAY BE INDIFFERENT TO LOVED ONES

CHARACTERISTIC DRAGGING PAINS

BETTER FOR VIGOROUS EXERCISE

GREAT SENSITIVITY TO COLD

ABOVE *The* Sepia *homeopathic remedy is derived from cuttlefish ink.*

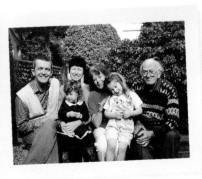

A classical homeopath gives one carefully selected remedy suited to your nature and symptoms. After taking the remedy, which may be one dose or a series of doses of one remedy, it is important to wait and see what changes take place. You will be asked to return for a further appointment so that the action of the remedy can be assessed. Sometimes you will experience a worsening or intensification of some symptoms after taking a constitutional remedy. This "aggravation" can be considered as the remedy "kicking in," and it is usually short-lived; if it is not, contact your homeopath. Aggravation of symptoms is usually a good indication that the remedy is well chosen for you, and you will feel better afterward – it is therefore to be looked forward to!

Cure is measured not only by the degree to which symptoms are relieved but also by how you feel in all aspects of your physical, emotional, and mental health. Depending on the complexity of your medical history, the healing process may take place over some time. How often you need to see a homeopath will depend on the nature and history of your complaints.

Professional homeopathic practitioners study medical sciences along with an intensive and lengthy training in the philosophy and practice of homeopathy. The profession is self-regulating, and to gain a license the practitioner must fulfill many hours of supervised practice and pass rigorous exams. Physicians who practice homeopathy may have had less training in homeopathy than professional homeopaths.

There are some variations in training and methods. If for any reason you are unsure about a doctor's or practitioner's homeopathic qualifications, it is always advisable to ask.

COMBINING WITH OTHER THERAPIES

There is a large and ever-increasing number of therapies available to those seeking to improve their health, including massage, acupuncture, psychotherapy, aromatherapy, Chinese herbalism, nutrition, and other alternative healing methods. There are no strict rules about using more than one at a time, but certain therapies may conflict with, or complement, each other. Homeopathy is an "energetic" form of medicine, because the remedies act on a person's vital energy. Therapies that may complement homeopathy are massage, psychotherapy, diet and nutrition, physiotherapy, osteopathy, and cranial osteopathy. Therapies that use other substances, such as herbalism and aromatherapy, may interfere with the action of homeopathic medicines.

Acupuncture and reflexology also stimulate the vital energy, but

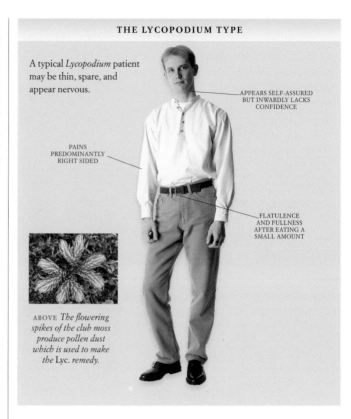

THE LYCOPODIUM TYPE

A typical *Lycopodium* patient may be thin, spare, and appear nervous.

APPEARS SELF-ASSURED BUT INWARDLY LACKS CONFIDENCE

PAINS PREDOMINANTLY RIGHT SIDED

FLATULENCE AND FULLNESS AFTER EATING A SMALL AMOUNT

ABOVE *The flowering spikes of the club moss produce pollen dust which is used to make the* Lyc. *remedy.*

on a somewhat different basis than homeopathy. If more than one energetic therapy is used at the same time it becomes difficult to know which one has helped, which may confuse the progress of longer term, constitutional treatment. If one method is succeeding, it is best to stay with it.

CAUTION

If you have an acute illness following constitutional treatment by your homeopath, do not try to treat yourself before you have consulted your homeopath.

COMBINING WITH CONVENTIONAL DRUGS

If you are on any form of regular medication, you should consult your physician and your homeopath before making any changes. Homeopathy can often work con currently with conventional medicine.

BELOW *Consult both your physician and homeopath before combining traditional medicine with homeopathic remedies.*

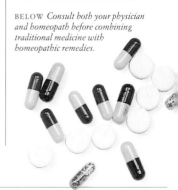

PROFESSIONAL CASE-TAKING

During the first consultation, the homeopath is taking your case. The complete constitutional picture includes important mental and physical characteristics. You may have a specific complaint, such as migraine headaches, but any other problems are equally significant, as well as how you are generally and in relation to your environment. You will be asked to talk about any problems you may experience. Here are some examples of the kind of information the homeopath will be interested in:

- What is difficult, problematic, causes stress in your life – whether from situations at home, in the work or study environment, or in relationships. How you react in stressful situations. This includes any fears, anxieties, or worries.

- Important or significant past events that were stressful, and how; whether or not the onset of any physical problems can be traced to that time.

- Weaknesses in the functioning of the mind, such as confusion, lack of ability to concentrate, or loss of memory.

- Areas of weakness in the body, where problems tend to occur – such as tendency to headaches, swollen glands, asthma, constipation, menstrual difficulties; how often, when they occur, what they feel like, what kinds of pain or other sensations accompany the complaints.

- Body temperature generally, whether you feel unusually hot or cold. How much perspiration and where.

Location	Sensation	
		Jackie Jones Date: 6·7·97
		114 Spratts Lane
		London E4 1BD Tel: 0171 876 3842
		Date of birth 12·3·60
HEAD	PAIN	Sensation as if a nail was being driven into the back of my skull
HEAD	TENSION	Feels very tight across forehead
STOMACH	STONE	Feel I have a stone sitting at the base of my stomach, it won't move
THROAT	LUMP	Always feel I have to swallow, it's as if there's something stuck in my throat and I can't get rid of it.
MIND	GRIEF	My brother was killed in a car crash last year. I can't stop crying and I think about him all the time. He was my favourite brother and we were very close. I didn't get to say goodbye.

Observation	Rubrics
SIGHING	
WEEPING	

- Irregularities of sleep; recurrent dreams or nightmares.

- Whether you feel better or worse in different environments, such as at the seaside, in the sunshine, or in closed rooms; or at certain times of day, or in a particular season of the year (modalities).

- Food and drink preferences – cravings and aversions.

- Medication taken, how much, when, and for what condition.

- Familial tendencies – diseases of parents, grandparents, siblings, etc., if known.

- Your level of energy generally and how you feel.

Guide to the Materia Medica

THE MATERIA MEDICA *is a compendium of the principal remedies used in homeopathy. The easiest way to find the entry that you are seeking is to consult the Repertory Index (see* pp. 126–133*), but in the Materia Medica each remedy is described in considerable detail to allow you to find and recognize the precise symptoms that you wish to treat. Each remedy's symptom picture (see p.19) is like a house. Some houses are large, some are smaller, but each one has its own particular characteristics, its own "architectural details." In the symptom picture house there are many different rooms, each of which represents a specific condition or complaint that you can treat with the remedy. Each room has its own individual details, but these in some way reflect the overall character of the house. For example, the "common cold" room of* Arsenicum *may at first sight seem quite similar to the same room in* Natrum muriaticum, *but the rooms are in keeping with their houses, and the overall character of each house is quite different.*

As you become acquainted with the Materia Medica, you will develop a feel for the remedies and for their symptom pictures as a whole, but the comprehensive information in this chapter helps the beginner to understand each remedy and the mental and physical symptoms that it will treat, and to compare each one with other remedies that might appear to treat the same symptoms.

ABOVE *Many remedies are derived from common plants such as white bryony.*

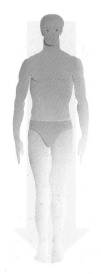

ABOVE *The healing process begins from the top of the body.*

RIGHT *Some symptom pictures include a strong aversion or desire for drink.*

How to use the Materia Medica

Once you have been referred to a particular remedy by the Repertory Index, the Materia Medica entry provides a complete profile of that remedy. A brief introduction gives the general history of the remedy.

This is followed by general indications of the remedy's symptom picture, as well as the accompanying mental state, modalities, and any particular desires or aversions to food or drink.

A Confirmation box, complete with symbols, gives the key characteristics of the symptom picture in a nutshell, and includes symbols for easy reference. A Complaints box lists the kinds of specific conditions that are best treated with this remedy.

In the Comparison of Remedies, you will find details of closely related symptom pictures for which other remedies might provide a better alternative.

Remedy name
This is the name of the remedy used by homeopaths and homeopathic pharmacies. In brackets you will see the abbreviated name as used in the Repertory Index. An introduction gives the source of the remedy and the method of homeopathic preparation, together with the symptoms for which it is prescribed.

Confirmation
The Confirmation box highlights the key symptoms that will confirm that you are considering the correct remedy for the particular case. Easily recognizable symbols provide an at-a-glance summary of the relevant symptoms and modalities.

Complaints
Each complaint is described with important details. It is very unlikely that every detail will describe your complaint, but if there are one or two symptoms that match strongly, you are on the right track. The complaints are organized roughly from the top of the body downward.

General indications
This tells you generally what the remedy treats: it is an overview of the remedy and its character. It tells you whether you are in the right house or not.

Modalities
These are what make the whole person better or worse. Use this section in conjunction with General indications. The modalities listed are possible, but not all modalities will apply to you.

Comparison of remedies
This will give you a quick reference to other remedies that have similarities, and that you might think appropriate for the complaint; it will help you to decide whether or not the "house" looks right. If you are unsure, refer to the whole remedy picture of another of these remedies.

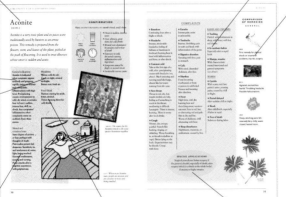

Mental and emotional state
This tells you about the "inner person," which is an important component of the illness. If your mental and emotional state is very different from the one described, you are most likely in the wrong house!

Food/drink
If you clearly have a strong desire for, or aversion to, a particular food or drink, you can use this to help you decide if a remedy is indicated. This symptom may not always be present.

Special applications
This box appears on certain entries, listing any specific uses, or circumstances that would indicate the remedy, such as surgery, traveling, and so forth.

Aconite

[ACON.]

Aconite is a very toxic plant and its juices were traditionally used by hunters as an arrow poison. This remedy is prepared from the flowers, stem, and leaves of the plant, picked at the peak of flowering. It is used to treat illnesses whose onset is sudden and acute.

CONFIRMATION

Plant: ACONITUM NAPELLUS *monk's-hood, wolf's-bane*

ONSET
sudden

THIRST
cold drinks

EMOTION
fearful

WORSE
at midnight

- *Onset is sudden, intense, acute*
- *Heat, dryness, great thirst for cold drinks*
- *Mental state dominated by anxiety and/or fear of death*
- *Exposure to cold, dry winds causing inflammation with high fever*
- *Symptoms caused by fright or mental shock*
- *Intolerable intense pains*

General indications

Aconite is indicated when symptoms appear suddenly and progress rapidly; pains are intense and unbearable; inflammations with high fever. Precipitating causes: overexposure to cold, dry wind, or extreme heat (of sun); sudden, intense fear, chill, or shock. Any symptoms/ inflammation when complaints come on suddenly from these causes.

Modalities

Worse: cold dry air; touch; at night, around midnight.
Better: rest; fresh air.

Food/drink

Desires: craving for acids, bitter, alcohol.
Thirst: burning thirst for cold drinks.

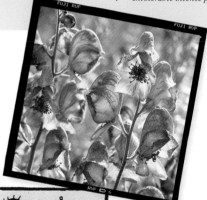

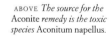

ABOVE *The source for the* Aconite *remedy is the toxic species* Aconitum napellus.

Mental and emotional state

Some degree of anxiety or fear, perhaps with thoughts of death. Pain makes person feel desperate. Sensitivity to, and intolerance of, noise, light, being touched. Extreme restlessness, tossing and turning. Panic attacks after a frightful experience, with palpitations.

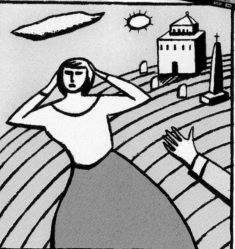

LEFT *When in an* Aconite *state, people are anxious and are sensitive to noise and being touched.*

COMPLAINTS

❖ **Emotions**
Continuing fears after a fright or shock.

❖ **Headache**
Intense, intolerable headache; feeling of fullness or heaviness in forehead; burning heat in head with inflammation and fever, or after shock.

❖ **Common cold**
Take at the first sign of a cold, after precipitating causes with headache (*see above*). Much sneezing and running nasal discharge, almost like hot water running from the nose.

❖ **Sore throat**
Throat is red, dry, hot; tonsils swollen and dry, feeling as if something is stuck in the throat; swallowing is difficult. Laryngitis. Thirst is intense, burning. Thirst is worse after iced drinks.

❖ **Cough**
Hoarse, dry, croupy, painful. Sounds like barking, ringing, or whistling. Worse breathing in, so breath is shallow or rapid. Better lying on the back. Expectoration may be bloody. Croup, with fever.

❖ **Earache**
Intense pain; noise is unbearable.

❖ **Toothache**
Intense, throbbing pain in teeth and head, with inflammation of the gums.

❖ **Digestive disorders**
Vomiting with fear; pain in stomach.

❖ **Colic**
With wind, distended abdomen, after fear.

❖ **Diarrhea**
From becoming overheated, or from exposure to cold wind. Nausea and sweating after diarrhea.

❖ **Fever**
High fever, with dry burning heat and drenching sweat; wants to uncover. Face is red, hot, or alternating red and pale. Skin is dry and hot. Waves of chilliness; chill alternating with heat.

❖ **Sleep disturbance**
Nightmares, insomnia, or restlessness, caused by fear.

BABIES AND CHILDREN

❖ **Teething**
Painful, with restlessness in sleep; with fever; with hot, red cheeks.

❖ **In newborn babies**
Especially after a rapid birth.

❖ **Mumps, measles**
With characteristic mental/emotional and general symptoms (*see above*).

WOMEN

❖ **Cystitis**
With scanty, red, hot, painful urine; pressing pains; caused by chill or fright.

❖ **Period delayed**
After sudden chill or fright.

❖ **Shock**
After childbirth, especially if labor is rapid.

❖ **Fear of death**
Before or during labor.

SPECIAL APPLICATIONS

Surgical procedures: before surgery, if the person is fearful, especially of death; after surgery (which is a shock to the whole body), if anxiety or fright remains.

COMPARISON OF REMEDIES

GENERAL

ARN.
First remedy for physical shock or trauma of accidents, injuries, surgery.

BELL.
Agitated, excited, less fearful. Throbbing headache. Possible hallucinations.

HEP.
Sharp, stitching pains felt intensely. Very chilly; wants closed, heated room.

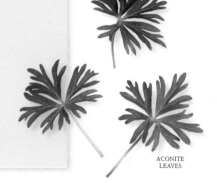

ACONITE LEAVES

31

Allium cepa

[ALL-C]

Prepared from the common onion, Allium cepa has long been used in traditional medicine for its healing properties. The fresh bulb is picked in the summer, then chopped and ground before mixing with alcohol to make a tincture. It is often used to treats colds and hayfever.

CONFIRMATION

Plant: ALLIUM CEPA *common onion*

WORSE
warm room

WORSE
damp cold
weather

- *Colds and hayfever*
- *Burning, watery eyes*
- *Bland discharge from nose*
- *Complaints from damp cold weather*
- *Worse for warmth and in the evenings*

WORSE
evening

BETTER
open air

General indications
Affects the mucous membranes of the upper respiratory tract. Colds in damp cold weather. Watery eyes as from chopping onions.

Mental and emotional state
No marked symptoms.

Modalities
**Worse: warm room; damp cold weather; evening.
Better: cold drinks while in a warm room; in a cool room; in open air.**

Food/drink
Desires: raw food (especially onions), vegetables.

COMPARISON OF REMEDIES

GENERAL

ACON.
Eye inflammations after exposure to cold, dry winds. Eyes are red hot and dry.

ARS.
Thin, watery, burning discharge from the nose that causes soreness of the upper lip. Generally restless; thirsty, but drinks in sips.

EUPH.
Bland discharge from the nose, with burning, acrid, stinging, watery eyes. Fits of sneezing.

GELS.
Slow onset of symptoms. Runny nose, with watery, acrid discharge, though nose feels blocked and dry. Feels as if hot water is running from the nose. Colds or flu in mild, damp, humid weather.

NAT-M.
Cold starts with forcible sneezing. Nose discharges are thin, and watery, or like white of an egg. Then nose becomes dry and blocked. Dryness alternates with fluent catarrh. May also have cold sores around the mouth or nose.

PULS.
Frequent sneezing, with yellow-green discharge from the nose. Symptoms change frequently. Person is clingy, seeks attention, and wants sympathy.

COMPLAINTS

❖ **Common cold**
Nasal catarrh with profuse, watery, acrid discharge, leaving sores on nostrils and upper lip; may be one-sided. Headache in forehead, with catarrhal congestion; forceful sneezing on getting up from bed.

❖ **Cough**
Hacking cough, worse for breathing in cold air; with sore throat and tickle in the larynx.

❖ **Eye complaints**
Eye inflammations: eyes burning, watery, with non-irritating, bland discharge.

❖ **Hayfever**
With the cold symptoms (*see above*); worse in late summer.

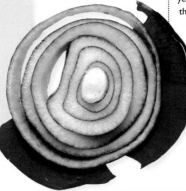

LEFT *The common red onion is the source for* Allium cepa.

Aloe

[ALOE]

The plant was traditionally used by the Greeks and Romans as a remedy for abdominal pain and disease. It is now used homeopathically to treat diarrhea, hemorrhoids and indigestion. Juice is extracted from the leaves of the aloe plant to make the tincture.

General indications
Affects lower abdomen and rectum. Burning pains. Symptoms of dysentery.

Modalities
Worse: early morning; hot weather; eating and drinking.
Better: cool open air; cold water; cold weather.

Food/drink
No marked desires or aversions.

CONFIRMATION

Plant: ALOE SUCCOTRINA *aloe*

WORSE
early morning

BETTER
cold weather

- *Sudden spluttering passing of loose stool*
- *Worse for eating and drinking*
- *Better for cold weather*

WORSE
eating/drinking

BETTER
open air

COMPARISON OF REMEDIES

DIARRHEA

ACON.
Diarrhea comes on suddenly, after being in a cold, dry wind, or as a result of a fright or shock. Stool may be green, like chopped herbs. Watery diarrhea in children on hot days. Also indicated for dysentery.

ARS.
A specific remedy for food poisoning. This person feels very chilly, but the diarrhea produces burning pains that feel better for heat. There may be burning pains in the stomach bowels, rectum, but all feels better for warmth, being wrapped up, or having warm applications. The burning discharges are quite thin and scanty not profuse. The person, though restless, feels quite anxious and exhausted – almost out of proportion to the illness. Burning thirst, with a desire to sip cold drinks. Over excitement.

PODO.
Noisy, gushing, explosive stool. Diarrhea with teething of babies and children.

COMPLAINTS

❖ **Indigestion**
Lower abdomen feels full and heavy, hot, bloated. Much wind presses down; wind is passed with burning pains. Diarrhea (*see below*).

❖ **Diarrhea**
Sudden urging, then passes gushing, watery stool. Weak feeling when passing wind, as if losing control of bowel. Unsure if stool or wind is passed. Stool is lumpy or watery with mucus. Passing stool is painful. Has to run to pass stool immediately after eating or drinking. Diarrhea after drinking beer; in early morning. Stools and urine pass at the same time; cannot pass one without the other.

❖ **Hemorrhoids**
Grapelike formation, burning pain, better in cold water.

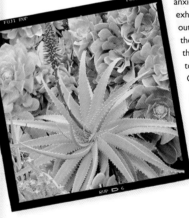

BELOW Aloe *is a tropical plant with succulent green leaves from the African continent.*

Antimonium tartaricum

[ANT-T.]

This remedy is made from heating oxide of antimony and acid potassium tartate; the crystals formed are dissolved to make the tincture. It is used to treat chest complaints, including whooping cough. In traditional medicine it was used as an expectorant and emetic.

CONFIRMATION

Mineral: TARTUS EMETICUS *tartar emetic*

BETTER sitting up

WORSE warm damp room

- *Inflammation of lungs, with great weakness*
- *Unproductive cough*
- *Vomiting*
- *Rattling in chest*

General indications
Affects mucous membranes of bronchi and lungs. Useful in cases of gradual, progressive weakness. Great accumulation of mucus with coarse rattling in the chest, where much would be expectorated, but patient is unable to expel it. Cold sweat, and great sleepiness.

Modalities
Worse: warm room; dampness. Better: sitting up; coughing up mucus (which is difficult).

Food/drink
Desires: acids, especially apples, which disagree; wants cold water – little amounts but often.

Mental and emotional state
Because of weakened state, patient is apathetic or easily annoyed, and wants to be alone. Child whines when touched.

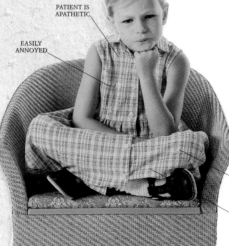

ABOVE *The source for* Antimonium tartaricum *is tartar emetic. It is a very poisonous substance.*

PATIENT IS APATHETIC

EASILY ANNOYED

WHINES WHEN TOUCHED

WANTS TO BE LEFT ALONE

RIGHT *A patient with* Antimonium tartaricum *characteristics wishes to be left alone and whines if touched.*

COMPLAINTS

GENERAL

❖ **Whooping cough, cough**
Loud, rattling cough. Shortness of breath as if suffocating. Chest is full but the person is too weak to raise expectoration. Cough followed by vomiting. Child arches back with cough. With a sore throat, tickle in throat excites the cough; swallowing is painful or impossible. With a fever, the face is pale, bluish, cold, covered with sweat.

❖ **Nausea**
With weakness and cold sweat.

❖ **Fever**
Copious, cold, clammy sweat.

BABIES

❖ **Breathing**
Inability to breathe in a newborn infant.

❖ **Whooping cough**
(*see above*).

DROS.
The chest feels tight and constricted rather than full of mucus. Cough from tickling sensation in the larynx. Fits of deep rapid barking or choking cough. Cough is painful, so person holds the sides of the chest to support the movement. Mood is irritable or restless. Whooping cough with nosebleeds and cold sweat. Symptoms are worse around midnight and from heat and better from open air.

HEP.
Barking and choking cough. Person is much worse from cold of any kind – cold air, cold drinks, the least draft of air. Person cries from pain before the cough. Much rattling in the chest, person brings up a lot of loose yellow phlegm, with difficulty. Emotionally touchy, and oversensitive to any external influence. Intense sharp pains mark this remedy.

IP.
Cough with nausea; also vomiting after cough without nausea. Person is thirstless, or the cough is relieved by drinking cold drinks. Suffocative, constant, and violent cough with inability to bring up phlegm. Nosebleeds from cough with nauseous feeling.

SPONG.
Extreme dryness of mucous membranes. Cough is dry, painful, and rasping. There is no rattling of mucus in the chest, no expectoration, or phlegm. Wakes from sleep, feeling suffocated and anxious. Sweet foods or drinks tickle the throat, warm drinks relieve. Complaints after exposure to cold, dry weather. If *Acon.* fails, try *Spongia*, particularly in cases of croup.

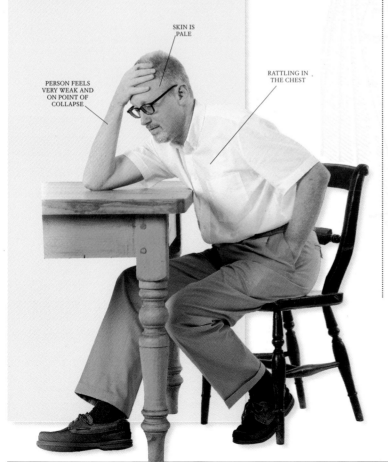

SKIN IS PALE

PERSON FEELS VERY WEAK AND ON POINT OF COLLAPSE

RATTLING IN THE CHEST

LEFT *A key symptom of the* Antimonium tartaricum *picture is apathy and lethargy.*

Apis mellifica

[APIS]

Since ancient time the honey bee has provided humans with a number of medicinal treatments, including remedies for ulcers, burns, and skin inflammations. The homeopathic remedy is prepared from the whole bee, including the poisonous sting. It is used to treat stings and bites, allergies, and inflammations.

CONFIRMATION

Insect: APIS MELLIFICA *honey bee*

WORSE
any heat

WORSE
touch

THIRST
absent

BETTER
open air

- *Heat, shiny redness, and swelling*
- *Lack of thirst*
- *Stings and bites, allergies, inflammations*
- *Burning stinging pains, better for cool, worse for warmth or heat*

General indications
Pains are characteristically burning, stinging, and prickly. Complaints are right-sided, or start on the right side and move to the left. Affected parts of the body are swollen, with a shiny red color; symptoms develop rapidly. The person is restless and sensitive to touch. Hot, but not thirsty. Allergic reactions.

Mental and emotional state
Fearful, tearful, irritable, excitable, busy, jealous, "touchy." Child does not want to be touched.

Modalities
Worse: heat of any kind – room, weather, fire, drinks, bath, or bed; touch or pressure. Better: cool air, cool bathing.

Food/drink
Aversions: drinks and water.

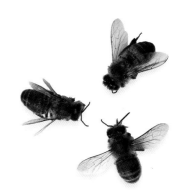

ABOVE *The honey bee is the source for* Apis mellifica. *The whole bee, including the sting, is used.*

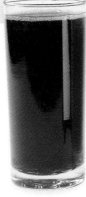

BEER

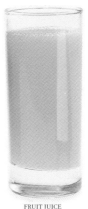

COLA

FRUIT JUICE

LEFT *The symptoms of the* Apis *remedy picture include an aversion to all kinds of drinks and water including fruit juice, alcohol and soft drinks.*

COMPLAINTS

❖ Emotions
Continuing fears after a fright or shock.

❖ Eye complaints
Puffy or red about eyes; conjunctiva bright red, puffy. Burning stinging pains. Hot tears.

❖ Earache
External ear is red, inflamed, and sore; stinging pains. Redness and swelling of both ears.

❖ Tonsillitis
Throat swollen inside and out. Tonsils swollen, fiery, and red or purplish, with a stinging pain when swallowing. Throat is better for cold drinks.

❖ Cystitis
Retention of urine. Burning pain and soreness occurs at the end of urination. Urine scanty, highly colored.

❖ Shingles (herpes zoster)
Swelling, with burning and stinging pains. Large vesicles come out in cold weather. Worse for warmth, better for cold applications.

❖ Hives, allergies
Any allergic reaction producing swelling, redness, and heat. Skin is rosy, shiny, red, sensitive, sore and/or dry, hot, swollen. Spots or large areas of raised skin (urticaria) that is rough and/or stinging. Face is red, hot, swollen, puffy; or waxy, pale, and puffy.

❖ Insect bites, stings
Effects of any sting or bite that leaves a red, shiny, swollen hot patch on the skin. Itches, burns, or stings that feel hot and are better for cold applications and worse for any heat.

❖ Joint pains
Joints feel bruised; red, shiny, swollen, with burning and stinging pains; worse for heat.

❖ Fever
Burning heat; heat alternating with chill; thirstless during fever, thirst during chill; wants to uncover; one part is hot, while another is cold.

CHILDREN

❖ Measles
Rash slow to emerge. With characteristic *Apis* general, mental, fever, and skin symptoms.

❖ Mumps
With characteristic *Apis* general and mental symptoms.

MEN

❖ Prostate
Enlarged prostate, with pain during urination.

PERSON IS
IRRITABLE AND
TEARFUL

PERSON IS
SENSITIVE
TO TOUCH

PATIENT HAS AN
AVERSION TO
DRINKS AND WATER

SYMPTOMS BEGIN
ON THE RIGHT
SIDE OF THE BODY

LEFT *Complaints for this remedy picture begin mainly on the right side of the body.*

ACON.
Inflammations after exposure to cold, dry wind, or symptoms that follow experience of sudden shock.

BELL.
Pains throbbing and pulsating rather than *Apis* burning and stinging. Dilated shining pupils; violent mental symptoms. Desire for lemons.

LACH.
Left-sided, no swelling, better for discharges, any discoloration (throat, skin, etc.) is dark red or purple.

LED.
Bites, stings, and puncture wounds that feel cold, but are better for cold application.

Argentum nitricum

[ARG-N.]

The remedy is made from pure crystals of silver nitrate dissolved in water. Arg-n. is used to treat nervous complaints and is a particularly useful remedy for those who suffer from exam nerves or stage fright. It was traditionally used to cauterize wounds.

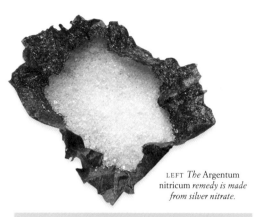

LEFT *The* Argentum nitricum *remedy is made from silver nitrate.*

General indications

Complaints that come on from excess mental exertion, such as intense studying, often with anticipatory anxiety about forthcoming events, such as exams, or speaking in front of an audience.
This may be accompanied by trembling, weakness, and nervousness. Person is restless and impulsive, and will be very hurried in manner, while speaking, walking, or waiting.
There may be a craving for candy, but very soon after comes diarrhea that is sometimes like chopped spinach. Warm-blooded types, usually worse in hot stuffy rooms and better for fresh air.

Mental and emotional state

Impulsive, hurried, nervous, fearful; dreads ordeals; fears something evil will happen; fear of crowds, tall buildings; claustrophobia.

Modalities

Worse: anxiety, anticipation of exams, public performance, mental strain; eating and drinking; sugar/candies causes diarrhea.
Better: company; cold (air or water); wind blowing on the face.

Food/drink

Desires: salt, salty foods, sugar (which make the person feel worse); cold drinks.
Aversions: candies, cheese.

RIGHT *The* Arg-n. *remedy picture is characterized by a strong reaction to candies.*

CONFIRMATION

Mineral: SILVER NITRATE *devil's stone, hellstone*

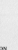

SENSATION
feels warm

THIRST
cold drinks

DESIRE AVERSION
candy

BETTER
open air

- *Numerous anxieties, particularly before important events, causing restlessness, hurriedness, impulsive behavior*
- *Sugar/candies are craved though they cause distention, diarrhea, and loud belching and flatulence*
- *Warm-blooded people with a craving for fresh air*

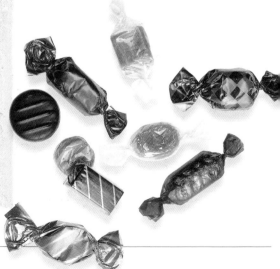

COMPLAINTS

❖ Emotional problems
Acute fear of exams, ordeals, performance; anxiety before these occasions. Hyperactivity in children.

❖ Headache
Nervous headache, feels as if head is in a vise. Headache ends in vomiting. Migraine.

❖ Eye complaints
Aching tired feeling in the eyes (from overwork); better for closing or pressing them. Acute conjunctivitis: inner corners of eyes swollen and red; copious, purulent discharge.

❖ Sore throat
Pain: feels as if a splinter is lodged in the throat. Laryngitis before public speaking.

❖ Digestive disorders
Loss of appetite; good appetite but all food disagrees.

❖ Stomach ulcers
Pain ulcerating. Pain in a small spot, which radiates in all directions; ulcer worse for eating cold food; eating improves the nausea but makes stomach pain worse.

❖ Flatulence
Abdomen distended with flatulence and belching loud and explosive, upward and downward.

❖ Diarrhea, constipation
Diarrhea from emotions, eating candies; constipation alternating with diarrhea (Irritable Bowel Syndrome).

❖ Trembling, weakness
Trembling hands; weakness in arms and legs; twisting in calf muscle. With emotional problems or other complaints.

CHILDREN

❖ Hyperactivity
Child is extremely impulsive, never thinking before acting. Episodes may be preceded by anticipating an important event, or exam.

COMPARISON OF REMEDIES

FOR ANTICIPATORY ANXIETY

GELS.
Exam nerves. Fear before an exam or ordeal causes the person to be quiet, or feel paralyzed. Trembling weakness or forgetfulness from overexcitement. These emotions accompany a nervous, painless diarrhea with yellow or green stool.

LYC.
Chilly person, lacking self-confidence, but dictatorial at home. Desire for candy, which does not affect the person adversely as in Arg-n. Worse 3–4 a.m. and 4–8 p.m. Anxiety may be felt in the stomach, with loss of appetite, or eating a little causes a feeling of fullness. Tending to have constipation rather than diarrhea.

BELOW *Anxiety about appearing in public is a key symptom of the Arg-n. remedy picture.*

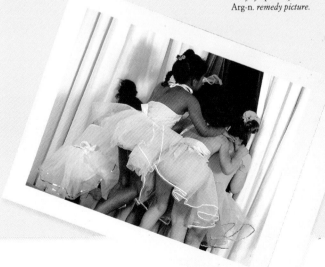

Arnica

[ARN.]

Also known as leopard's bane, Arnica *grows in the mountains of Europe and in Siberia. The remedy is made from the whole plant, including the root. It is used homeopathically as a first aid remedy, particularly to treat shock and trauma.* Arnica *cream is also available for application to bruises and swellings.*

CONFIRMATION

Plant: ARNICA MONTANA *leopard's bane, fall-kraut, mountain tobacco, sneezewort*

SENSATION
feels cold

WORSE
touch

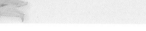

BETTER
open air

- *Trauma – to either whole body or part of it*
- *Mechanical injuries*
- *Fear of touch, fear of being approached*
- *Sore, bruised feeling*

General indications

This is the first remedy to think of in case of trauma, injury, and any case of major or minor physical stress, such as car accident, broken bones, falls, surgical procedures. Person feels sore, aching, bruised externally and/or internally, even the bed feels too hard. In cases of bruised tissue or joints, *Arn.* can help to reduce swelling and inflammation.

Modalities

Worse: touch, jarring; after childbirth; during labor; overexertion; after sleep, eating.
Better: lying down, with head low; open air; cold bathing; changing position.

Food/drink

Desires: sour drinks, alcohol, beer.
Aversions: food, meat; tobacco, smoking.

CAUTION

Arnica cream is also available, which can help to speed the curative process after bruising. However, it must not be applied to broken skin.

Mental and emotional state

Person may be generally fearful of being approached (even, and especially, by the physician), or may be anxious about someone touching the injury – a characteristic reaction is the person saying nothing is wrong, wanting to be left alone.

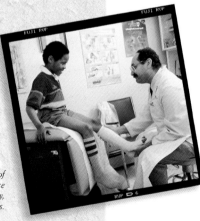

RIGHT Arnica *is one of the main remedies to use after a traumatic injury, especially broken bones.*

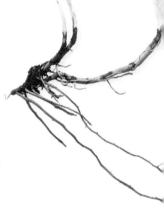

COMPLAINTS

❖ Emotional problems
After mental or physical shock or trauma.

❖ Headache
Migraine from injury to head. Face hot, while limbs cold. *Arn.* can be given for any blow to the head.

❖ Loss of vision
After blow to the eye.

❖ Nosebleed
After blow to the nose. Nosebleed with whooping cough.

❖ Toothache, bleeding gums
Pains in the teeth after head injury or tooth extraction. Gums bleeding after dental work, tooth extraction.

❖ Skin bruising, rash
Easily bruised; every hurt causes bruising; measles. *Arnica* cream can be applied to local bruising but should not be applied to broken skin.

❖ Injuries
Falls, blows, bruises, dislocation, sprains, or strains, of muscles, joints, soft tissues, bone. Overexertion, exhaustion from too much sports or exercise. The whole person, or one part, feels bruised, aching, sore, as if beaten. Hemorrhages, black and blue marks.

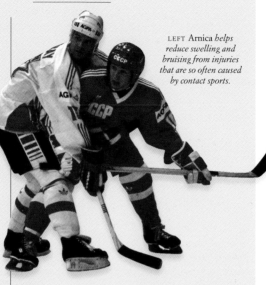

LEFT Arnica *helps reduce swelling and bruising from injuries that are so often caused by contact sports.*

SPECIAL APPLICATIONS
Before surgery, helps strengthen the system; after surgery, promotes recovery. Once there is recovery from the immediate trauma of surgery, other remedies may follow according to the nature of the surgery and more specific indications.

WOMEN

❖ Pregnancy
Threatened abortion from falls; soreness of whole body during pregnancy or labor; backache during pregnancy; after childbirth.

❖ Childbirth
Afterpains when breastfeeding; soreness after labor; labor weak and ceasing.

COMPARISON OF REMEDIES
FOR TRAUMA AND INJURY

ACON.
Person is fearful from a shock or fright.

BELL-P.
Deep tissue trauma when *Arn.* does not help.

HAM.
Bruised sore pains, worse for touch. Can be taken after *Arn.* where soreness and bruised feeling persists.

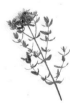

HYP.
Trauma is to nerves/nervous tissue; spinal injuries.

RHUS T.
After *Arn.* for sprains and strains of muscles or joints that are better for continued motion.

41

Arsenicum album

[ARS.]

A well-known poison, Arsenic is lethal in large doses. The homeopathic remedy is prepared by heating natural arsenides of iron, nickel, and cobalt, which are then diluted by trituration. It is used to treat digestive disorders and fevers. Arsenic was traditionally used to treat syphillis.

CONFIRMATION

Mineral: ARSENIC TRIOXIDE

BETTER
heat

SENSATION
feels cold

THIRST
cold drinks

- *Mood is anxious, despairing, fussy*
- *Chilly, yet burning pains that are relieved by heat*
- *Weak but restless; cannot find a comfortable place*
- *Very thirsty but drinks only in sips*
- *Worse 1–2 a.m.*

General indications

In cases of acute illness this remedy will affect the nervous system. Anxiety, restlessness; mucous membranes discharge thin, acrid, scanty fluids. The person is suddenly weak, and the degree of prostration seems out of proportion to the illness. The person is chilly and has burning pains, like hot needles, which feel better for hot applications. Digestion is affected, as if poisoned. Face is pale, with anxious expression, and covered with cold sweat. Specific for food poisoning.

Mental and emotional state

Oversensitive, fault finding, exacting, fussy. Expresses fear of death and great anxiety about health. Extreme restlessness; the person continually changes place or position; children want to be carried, do not settle, and do not want to be left alone.

Modalities

Worse: cold drinks, food, ice cream, air; after midnight, 1–2 a.m.; drinking; exertion. Better: warmth, heat; walking (moving) around; company.

Food/drink

Desires: warm drinks, food; olives or olive oil. Aversions: food; smell of food; cold. Thirst: very thirsty for cold or iced water, which is drunk in sips, but makes the person feel worse.

ABOVE *Highly toxic arsenic oxide provides the source for the* Ars. *remedy.*

BELOW *When in an* Ars. *state, the person is very anxious about his or her health and greatly fears death.*

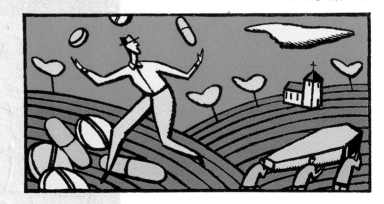

COMPLAINTS

❖ **Common cold**
Nose feels stopped up, yet produces a thin, watery, fluent, burning discharge causing soreness of the upper lip. Sneezing brings no relief; sneezing with irritating watery coryza.

❖ **Sore throat**
Throat feels swollen, constricted with burning pain.

❖ **Hayfever**
With characteristic *Ars.* general, mental, and emotional symptoms, and nose symptoms (*see above – Common cold*).

❖ **Cough**
Shortness of breath; must sit up. Wheezing. Cough alternately dry and loose, dry at night, person must sit up, worse for drinking. Little expectoration. Face bluish, with cold sweat and anxious expression.

❖ **Influenza**
With symptoms of cold, fever, and/or cough.

❖ **Digestive disorders**
Loss of appetite, or desire for sour things. Cannot bear sight or smell or thought of food. Burning pain better for sweet milk; heartburn; vomiting. Breath foul. Gnawing burning pains, in the abdomen, better for heat. Violent pains; cannot get comfortable, rolls around, with anguish.

❖ **Painful vomiting**
Symptoms of food poisoning, with nausea, vomiting, diarrhea. Craves ice-cold water, which is immediately vomited. Digestive problems when traveling abroad.

❖ **Diarrhea**
Copious, burning, with undigested food; causes weak feeling. Stool green, gray, light; offensive, putrid, watery.

❖ **Urine retention**
Urine scanty, burning.

❖ **Skin hives, rash**
Hives from eating shellfish. Measles: vesicles that burn violently. With characteristic *Arsenicum* general, mental, fever symptoms.

❖ **Fever**
Externally cold, but internally burning hot. Sensitive to cold, but better in the open air. Chills, shaking; craves hot drink during chill. Heat as if burning in veins. High fever. Sweat with great thirst, breathing difficulties, prostration; feeling icy cold or burning heat. Intermittent fever; yellow fever.

WOMEN

❖ **Urine retention**
After childbirth, as if bladder were paralyzed.

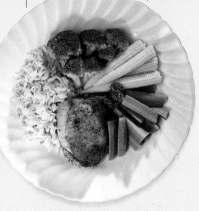

RIGHT Digestive symptoms include an aversion to the sight, smell, or even the thought of food.

Belladonna

[BELL.]

*Commonly known as deadly nightshade,
Belladonna was traditionally used by witches
in their magical potions during the Middle
Ages. To make the homeopathic remedy, the
whole plant is gathered at the time of flowering,
then macerated and soaked in alcohol from
which a tincture is made.*

General indications

Affects nerves, brain,
circulation, mucous
membranes. Sudden and
violent onset.
Inflammations with
burning heat, dryness,
bright redness.
Inflammations of one part
of the body with redness
or streaks of red. Pupils
dilated; eyes have staring,
sparkling quality. Hot
body parts, discharges.
Severe neuralgic pain,
comes and goes quickly.
Pain throbbing, sharp,
cutting, shooting. Spasms
and twitching. Right-
sided symptoms. Suits
vigorous people, like
children, who become ill
suddenly and violently.

Mental and emotional state

Senses acute; wildly
delirious, excited, noisy,
cries out. Restless; biting,
striking; hallucinates
monsters; fears imaginary
things. "An angel when
well, a devil when sick."

Modalities

Worse: sun's heat; drafts,
or wet and cold on head;
light, noise, jarring
(because nerves are
affected); touch, motion.
Doesn't like to look at
bright shining objects.
Better: light covering, rest
in bed; dark room;
standing or sitting erect;
warm room.

Food/drink

Desires: lemonade,
lemons, beer, cold drinks.
Aversions: coffee, drinks;
smell of food, cooked
food.
Thirst: for cold water,
except during fever.

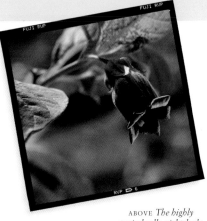

ABOVE *The highly
toxic deadly nightshade
species is the source for
the* Belladonna *remedy.*

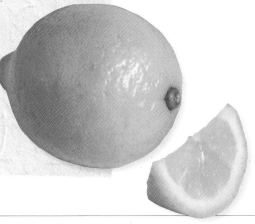

LEFT *Symptoms include
a thirst for lemonade or
a desire for lemons.*

COMPLAINTS

❖ **Common cold**
With headache (*see below*), dry, red, sore throat, and swollen glands.

❖ **Headache**
Throbbing, hammering, bursting headache, worse for motion. Feels better for putting hand on head. Rolls head, pulls hair. Headache from overexposure to the sun.

❖ **Eye complaints**
Red conjunctiva; photophobic. Bloodshot, burning, and dry; watering. Eye symptoms with common cold or fever.

❖ **Earache**
Painful inflammation of the middle ear, especially on right side. Pain causes delirium. Ears are red, hot, throbbing. Pain extends from the ear into the face.

❖ **Sore throat**
Throat dry and hot. Tonsillitis, especially on right side; may have red streaks. Swallowing difficult. Laryngitis.

❖ **Cough**
Tickling, short, dry, barking. Whooping cough, with pain in stomach before attack. Child cries before cough. Larynx very painful.

❖ **Digestive disorders**
Vomits everything. Abdomen distended and hot, worse for slightest touch (even of bedclothes).

❖ **Abscesses**
Skin is bright red, glossy, dry, and hot. With inflammation, fevers.

❖ **Sleep disturbance**
Jerks during sleep; nightmares; sees frightful things on closing eyes, for example, monsters on the bed.

❖ **Fever**
High fever, with internal coldness. Hot head with cold limbs. No thirst during fever. Face: fiery red, turgid, hot; or pale and red alternately.

WOMEN

❖ **Mastitis**
With pain, throbbing, redness, streaks radiating from the nipples; breast heavy, hard, and red.
❖ **Presurgery:** before curettage.

CHILDREN

❖ **Measles**
With bright-red rash. With characteristic *Belladonna* general, mental, and fever symptoms. Any childhood illness with characteristic symptoms of *Belladonna*.

SPECIAL APPLICATIONS

Sunstroke, with headache and fever.

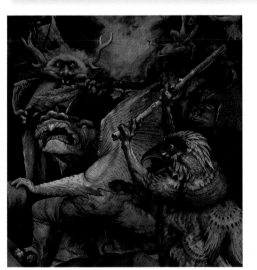

LEFT *The* Bell. *mental state is often characterized by delirium and people may experience hallucinations.*

COMPARISON OF REMEDIES

FOR FEVER

ACON.
Sudden onset; dry, burning heat, more anxious and fearful of death. General inflammation. More thirsty during a fever.

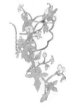

BRY.
Slow onset; dryness everywhere. Person must keep still, worse for the least movement.

Bellis perennis

[BELL-P.]

Known as the English arnica, Bellis perennis has been used since the Middle Ages to treat wounds. It is still used for this purpose, especially for treating internal wounds after accidents or surgery. The remedy is prepared from the whole flowering plant, which is macerated and steeped in alcohol to make the tincture.

CONFIRMATION

Plant: BELLIS PERENNIS *English daisy, woundwort*

WORSE
touch

WORSE
chilled

BETTER
movement

- *Internal bruising and injuries after accidents or surgery*
- *After abdominal surgery*
- *Worse if becomes chilled while hot*

General indications
A great trauma remedy, for deep (internal) trauma or septic wounds, especially of abdominal and pelvic organs, after major surgical operations. Therefore good for childbirth, particularly cesarian births. Tumors from injury. Much worse on becoming chilled when hot. Complaints may follow suddenly becoming chilled, such as swimming in very cold water, or drinking cold drinks while overheated.

Mental and emotional state
No marked symptoms.

Modalities
Worse: injury, touch; cold baths or drinks; warm bed.
Better: continued motion; cold applied locally.

Food/drink
Desires: meat, onions, pickles, vinegar.

ABOVE *The common daisy has great healing powers and is the source for* Bellis perennis, *used to treat internal wounds.*

RIGHT Bellis perennis *is one of the main remedies for the treatment of abdominal wounds after surgery.*

COMPLAINTS

❖ **Emotions**

Continuing fears after a fright or shock.

❖ **Injuries, wounds**

Surgical incisions that become infected. Hemorrhages. Tissues surrounding injury are very sore and cannot tolerate touch or cold bathing. Swelling of tissues remains after treatment with *Arn*.

WOMEN

❖ **Injuries**

Injuries to breasts and genitalia. Injuries to breasts where a bump or lump remains after the initial bruising has cleared.

USE *BELL-P.* FOR
STRAINED
ABDOMINAL
MUSCLES

VARICOSE VEINS
ARE A COMMON
COMPLAINT
DURING
PREGNANCY

❖ **During pregnancy**

when there is difficulty walking due to straining of abdominal muscles, internal bruising of uterus by kicking of fetus or pressure on groin due to the weight of the fetus. Varicose veins in pregnancy, with characteristic modalities.

❖ **After childbirth**

when bearing down or labor pains remain, or when mechanical interference (e.g. forceps) have left internal pains. Uterus infected after childbirth or cesarian.

USE *BELL-P.* TO
RELIEVE BRUISING
OF THE UTERUS

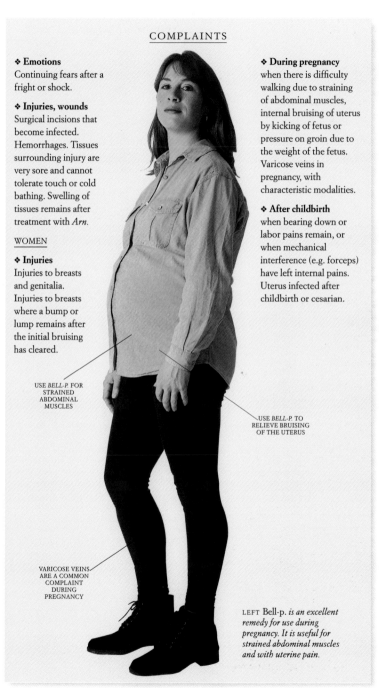

LEFT Bell-p. *is an excellent remedy for use during pregnancy. It is useful for strained abdominal muscles and with uterine pain.*

ARN.

First remedy to try in cases of shock/injury. Can precede *Bell-p.* Both *Arn.* and *Bell-p.* have bruised, sore feeling but *Bell-p.* affects especially deep abdominal tissues. Bruising of muscle, bone, skin, injuries of joints. Fatigue from overexertion. Mental state – denies the illness and wants to be left alone.

HAM.

Hemorrhages from injury, followed by prostration. Sore pains externally. Distension of veins.

HYP.

Injuries to nerve endings (fingers/toes/spine), resulting in shooting pains. Falls. After dental work if pain remains following needle injection.

STAPH.

Surgical wounds are painful, or become infected. Anger/indignation, or sense of invasion after surgery.

47

Bryonia

[BRY.]

Bryonia *has traditionally been used to treat such ailments as vertigo, melancholia, delirium, and gout. The root is taken before the plant flowers, then macerated and soaked in alcohol to make the tincture. It is used to treat illnesses that develop slowly with pain on any movement.*

CONFIRMATION

Plant: BRYONIA ALBA, *wild hops, black bryony*

WORSE
movement

THIRST
cold water

BETTER
open air

- *Dry, parched; thirsty for large quantities of water*
- *Worse for the least movement; better keeping still, holding the painful part*
- *Most symptoms worse for warmth, warm room; better for cool, open air*

General indications

Symptoms develop slowly, over a few days. Illness may begin after becoming chilled on a warm day, or when weather changes from cold to warm. Headaches with most complaints. Many parts of the body become extremely dry, especially mucous membranes. Every little movement is painful. Pains are bursting, sharp, or sore. Children do not want to be carried or lifted up. Slight exertion makes the person feel weak. Useful for injuries to joints – after *Arnica* – that are definitely worse when moving. Inflammation of serous membranes (membranes that line certain large cavities of the body, and surround organs – for example, lungs). Face is dark red, with dry, cracked lips.

Mental and emotional state

Irritable, ugly behavior. Wants to be quiet and left alone. A characteristic symptom is wanting to go home, even if the person is already there. Expresses concerns about business or money.

Modalities

Worse: anything that causes movement – bending forward, coughing, deep breathing, sneezing, eye movements, blinking; becoming hot in a hot room.
Better: pressure, lying on the painful part, keeping still; cool open air; wet weather; warm applications to inflamed part.

Food/drink

Desires: coffee, wine, acid drinks.
Aversions: coffee, rich food, fat, meat, milk.
Does not relish food.
Thirst: for large quantities of cold water, drunk infrequently.

ABOVE Bryonia *is prepared from the white bryony, a climbing plant.*

LEFT *When in a* Bryonia *state the person wishes to be quiet and left alone.*

COMPLAINTS

❖ **Headache**
Bursting, splitting headache, from forehead to the back of the head. Worse for any movement. Feels better for bending head backward or closing eyes. Pain begins in the morning, and gets worse during the day. Headache with constipation. Face dark red, hot, bloated. Dizziness. Sensitive scalp. Lips dry and cracked. Mouth dry, taste bitter. Tongue has white coating.

❖ **Common cold**
Cold begins in nose, with much sneezing and runny nose, watery, achy eyes and headache, then progresses to throat and larynx. Cough ends in vomiting.

❖ **Cough**
Dry, hard, painful cough. Brings up blood-streaked sputum. Sharp stitches in chest.

❖ **Influenza**
Headache (*see above*); achy limbs, cough, chest pain, with characteristic mental and general or fever symptoms.

❖ **Digestive disorders**
Bitter taste in the mouth. Dry mouth, with white coating on the tongue. Stomach sensitive to touch. Nausea and faintness when rising up from bed. Vomits bile and water immediately after eating. Cramping pain

relieved by drawing the knees up. Problems after overeating, especially meat. Abdomen very sore to touch. Distension and colic after eating. Sharp burning pain, worse for pressure, coughing, or breathing. Liver inflammation, appendicitis, peritonitis. Constipation, with large, dry, very hard stool, as if burned. Diarrhea in the morning: loose, painless stool, containing undigested food.

❖ **Fever**
Dry, burning heat. Hot head, red face. Cold to touch but hot internally. Sweating absent or profuse.

❖ **Joint Pains**
Injuries to joints (after *Arnica*). Red, swollen, hot. Inflammation of tissues, feels much worse for the least movement. Pains as if sprained. Heavy, weary, weak stiff feeling of limbs.

CHILDREN

❖ **Measles**
Undeveloped measles; spots are slow to develop. Measles with *Bryonia* characteristic mental and general symptoms, and hard, dry cough.

WOMEN

❖ **Breastfeeding**
Hot, painful, hard breasts, with pale red color. Worse for moving. Mastitis.

COMPARISON OF REMEDIES
FOR ACUTE INFLAMMATION

ACON.
Sudden onset. Very restless and fearful – thoughts of death.

ARS.
Extremely weak and restless; keeps moving; drinks little and often.

BELL.
Rapid, vigorous onset. Brain affected. Thumping headache, better for sitting up.

GELS.
Aching, heaviness, physical weakness. Not thirsty.

RHUS T.
Joint pains relieved by continued movement.

SPONG.
Feeling of suffocation. Croupy cough: barking, sawing. Whistling and wheezing respiration; compelled to sit up and bend forward. Starting from sleep.

RIGHT Bryonia *can be used to relieve acute, painful headaches.*

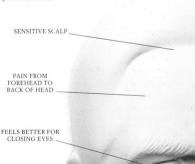

SENSITIVE SCALP

PAIN FROM FOREHEAD TO BACK OF HEAD

FEELS BETTER FOR CLOSING EYES

Calcarea carbonica

[CALC.]

This is one of the key homeopathic remedies and is used for a wide range of treatments. It is made from a fine layer of calcium carbonate found in the middle layer of the shell of the European edible oyster. It is a good remedy for children with slow development.

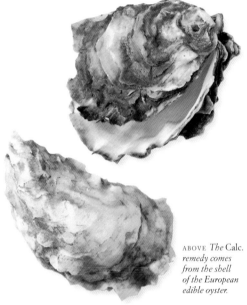

ABOVE *The* Calc. *remedy comes from the shell of the European edible oyster.*

General indications
This remedy is usually prescribed on the basis of constitutional symptoms and is one of the most important children's remedies. It affects assimilation of food and calcium metabolism in various ways. Useful for children who are late walking and talking, lack muscle tone, and tend to put on weight. Muscles become lax, flabby. They sweat easily, especially on the head during sleep. Complaints of teething children, with sour diarrhea. People who are susceptible to cold, or who sprain easily. Hands and feet tend to be cold and damp (clammy). Sour smells generally. Glands tend to enlarge. Perspires on the back of the head, especially during sleep.

Mental and emotional state
Children can be easily frightened, or offended, self-willed, fearful, or mischievous, obstinate. Learning is slow or methodical. Sensitive to criticism and dislikes being observed. Babies who are normally happy and content become more difficult when teething.

Modalities
Worse: cold, damp weather; physical or mental exertion; teething; milk. Better: dry climate.

Food/drink
Desires: boiled eggs, candies, milk, cold drinks, ice cream. May crave chalk, coal, or pencils. Aversions: milk, which upsets the stomach; meat, fat, rich food, slimy food.

CONFIRMATION

Mineral: CALCIUM CARBONATE
carbonate of lime, oystershell

SENSATION
chilly

WORSE cold
damp weather

WORSE
movement (exertion)

BETTER
dry climate

- *Chilly, sweaty, especially on head during sleep. Takes cold easily*
- *Easily frightened or obstinate*
- *Teething difficulties*
- *Sour sweat, stool*
- *Craving for candy and boiled eggs; worse for milk*

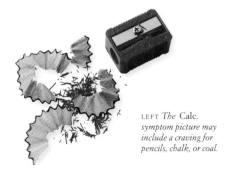

LEFT *The* Calc. *symptom picture may include a craving for pencils, chalk, or coal.*

COMPLAINTS

❖ **Common cold**
Cold comes on whenever the weather changes. Offensive yellow discharge from the nose. Lingering colds. Swelling of the nose and upper lip in children. Swollen glands.

❖ **Cough**
Dry cough, worse at night; able to expectorate in the morning, loose during the day. Hoarse throat without pain, worse in morning. Shortness of breath; tickling cough.

❖ **Digestive disorders**
Sour taste in the mouth. Indigestion, frequent sour belching, sour vomiting of curdled milk; milk upsets the stomach. Abdomen distended, large, and hard. Colic. Child feels better when constipated. Stool large and hard at first, followed by diarrhea containing undigested food.

❖ **Fever**
Chill with thirst; icy coldness in different parts of the body. Heat inside, cold to the touch. Head sweaty; night sweats.

❖ **Skin affections**
Small wounds do not heal.

RIGHT Calc. *is often used as a constitutional remedy for children.*

CHILDREN

Diarrhea with teething (*see* Children).

❖ **Sleep disturbance**
Nightmares in children, who cannot be quieted. Horrible vision on closing eyes.

WOMEN

❖ **Teething problems**
Sour-smelling, watery diarrhea, containing undigested food; worse after drinking milk.

❖ **Cradle cap**
Thick, foul milkcrusts, on the head.

❖ **Breastfeeding**
Overabundance of milk, which disagrees with the child. Too little milk; nipple cracked, ulcerated, tender.

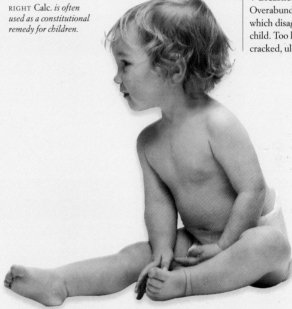

COMPARISON OF REMEDIES
GENERAL

CHAM.
Irritable and angry with pain; green diarrhea; child wants to be carried.

LYC.
Colicky, windy babies; tend to be worse 4–8 p.m. and after midnight.

PULS.
Clingy, wants sympathy and attention, worse in a warm room, needs fresh air.

SIL.
Sensitive, anxious, and fearful. Chilly, better for warmth. Perspiration can be offensive, stool difficult to pass. Abscesses, boils, ulcers, and pustules. Promotes the expulsion of splinters from under the surface of the skin.

Calendula

[CAL.]

The homeopathic remedy is made from the fresh flowering tops and leaves of the marigold plant. It is generally used topically in the form of cream, tincture, ointment, or oil. It is an essential component of any first aid kit and may be used to bathe and sterilize wounds and grazes.

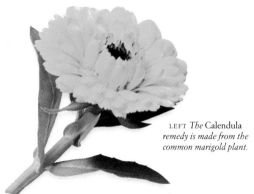

LEFT *The* Calendula *remedy is made from the common marigold plant.*

General indications

Acts as an antiseptic, and promotes rapid and healthy new skin growth of tissue. Superficial open wounds – cuts, tears, lacerations, burns, or very painful wounds. Hemorrhages after tooth extractions. Helps to prevent suppuration.

The tincture is made with a high percentage of alcohol, and may sting if used undiluted. Make up solutions as follows to promote faster healing:
• Cuts, wounds and grazes: dilute 10 drops in a bowl of warm water to clean the damaged area before applying dressings.
• Postnatal situations: appropriate for postnatal use in healing after episiotomy. Either bathe the area as above, or add 10–20 drops of tincture to the bath.
• As a mouthwash: after tooth extraction, or with mouth ulcers, dilute 5 drops in half a glass of water.

• As an eyebath: in cases of conjunctivitis, *Calendula* **will clean the area and soothe the eyes. Use 1–2 drops in an eyebath of warm water.**
• To clean and dry up blisters after they have burst, and promote new skin growth.

Mental and emotional state
No marked symptoms.

Modalities
No marked modalities.

Food/drink
No marked desires or aversions.

BELOW Calendula's *antiseptic qualities make it ideal for use on cuts and wounds.*

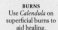

MARIGOLD PETALS

CALENDULA CREAM

BURNS
Use *Calendula* on superficial burns to aid healing.

WOUNDS
Calendula helps prevent wounds from becoming infected.

NEW TISSUE
Scar tissue will form more quickly over cuts if *Calendula* is used.

Calendula *cream or ointment may be applied directly to affected areas, and is useful in the treatment of diaper rashes, irritated, broken, or cracked and dry skin. Use cream or ointment when you wish to keep the area moist and supple.*

• *To soften cracked nipples*
• *To soften the perineum after childbirth*
• *To help superficial burns to heal more quickly*
• *To allow grazes to heal without skin becoming dry and scarring*
• *As a general soothing cream for dry hands after hard labor, e.g. in the garden, or after using tools*

COMPARISON OF REMEDIES
GENERAL

ARN.
Cream applied externally: bruises. Do not apply to open wounds.

CANTH.
Take internally for second-degree burns with violent pains, rawness, and smarting.

CAUST.
Take internally for third-degree burns, scalds, or chemical burns. Burning pain with blisters. Burns that are slow to heal.

HAM.
Cream, or diluted tincture, applied externally to varicose veins and hemorrhoids.

RHUS T.
Applied externally to soothe sprains or strained muscles. With pain on initial movement, but improvement on continued motion.

URT-U.
Cream applied externally to first-degree burns, uticaria, nettle rash. Worse after bathing, violent exercise. Violent itching. Burning, stinging pains; local burns; sunburn.

BELOW *Soothing* Calendula *cream may be applied directly to affected areas.*

COMPLAINTS

❖ **Bleeding gums**
After dental work: use diluted tincture to rinse mouth.

❖ **Cuts/wounds**
Characteristic *Cal.* general symptoms.

❖ **Burns**
In the later stages of healing, after first- or second-degree burns, after blisters have burst. Sunburn. *Cal.* will promote new skin growth.

❖ **Rash**
Calendula cream helps to reduce the irritation of eczema: soothes rashes, heals raw and cracked areas. *Eczema should always be treated constitutionally by a professional homeopath.*

CHILDREN

❖ **Diaper rash**
Apply cream to clean and dry areas.

WOMEN

❖ **Childbirth**
Before childbirth apply cream to perineum to soften skin; after childbirth use diluted tincture to speed healing of episiotomy or tears, or cesarian incision.

❖ **Breastfeeding**
Apply cream to cracked nipples between feeds; remove traces of cream before feeding.

PROMOTES NEW SKIN GROWTH

HEALS RAW CRACKED AREAS

SOOTHES RASHES

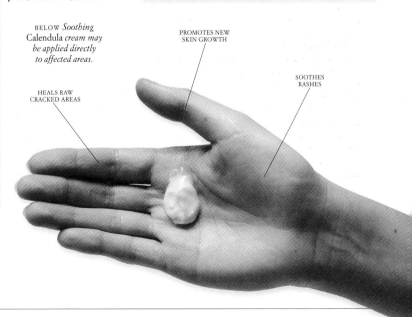

Cantharis

[CANTH.]

Cantharis *comes from the blister beetle or Spanish fly, an insect found all over southern Europe. The whole dried insect is ground to a fine powder to make the remedy. Traditionally used as an aphrodisiac and to treat warts,* Cantharis *is used homeopathically to treat illnesses with burning symptoms.*

CONFIRMATION

Insect: LYTTA VESICATORIA *Spanish fly*

ONSET
sudden

WORSE
touch

- *Burning pains*
- *Urinary/sexual organs*
- *Complaints where onset is rapid*
- *Violent inflammations*
- *Unquenchable thirst*

General indications
Affects urinary and sexual organs. Onset is rapid and intense, inflammations are violently acute. Pains are burning. Valuable for healing burns and scalds. Right side most affected.

Modalities
**Worse: urinating, touch, cold drinks, coffee; the sound of water.
Better: warmth, rest, rubbing, lying quietly on the back.**

Food/drink
**Aversions: food, drinks, water, tobacco.
Thirst: unquenchable.**

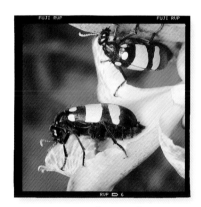

ABOVE Cantharis *is made from Spanish fly, a bright green European beetle.*

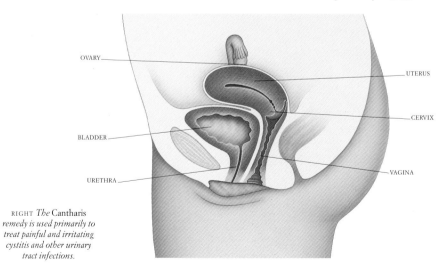

OVARY

UTERUS

CERVIX

BLADDER

VAGINA

URETHRA

RIGHT *The* Cantharis *remedy is used primarily to treat painful and irritating cystitis and other urinary tract infections.*

COMPARISON OF REMEDIES
FOR CYSTITIS

ACON.

Cystitis with scanty, red, hot painful urine. Caused by sudden chill, shock, or frightening experience.

APIS

Burning and stinging pains during urination; thirstless; better for cold bathing; mood angry, tearful, busy, fidgety.

ARS.

Retention of urine, as if bladder were paralyzed, after childbirth. Scanty urine with burning pain. Person is generally chilly, anxious, restless, or overly fussy; thirsty for cold drinks that are drunk as sips, worse for cold, better for warmth and company.

CAUST.

Cystitis with constant urge to urinate and difficulty in passing urine. Burning in urethra during urination, then pain in the bladder after having passed a few drops. Urine may leak on coughing or laughing.

LYC.

Urine retention, urine slow in coming, must strain to pass urine. Copious urination at night. Pressing feeling in bladder and abdomen.

PULS.

Scanty urine with strong ammonia smell. Burning pain during and after urination, at the opening of the urethra. Bland, yellow-green discharges. Tendency to affections of mucous membranes.

SEP.

Cystitis with pain as if cutting like knives. Constant urge to urinate; urine is milky, burning, bloody. Urine may leak on coughing or laughing, due to laxity of pelvic floor muscles.

STAPH.

Cystitis with burning during and after urination, but pain when not urinating distinguishes this remedy. Cause may be oversensitivity of bladder after love-making or coition. Pressure upon bladder, as if it did not empty. Copious and involuntary urination especially on coughing. Less violent pain than *Canth*.

COMPLAINTS

❖ **Cystitis**
Constant, intolerable urge to urinate. Only a few drops are passed at a time, with cutting, burning pain. The urine burns, scalds, and may contain blood. Kidney region is sensitive. Violent pain in bladder, intolerable straining; with pains before, during, and after urinating. A notable symptom is unquenchable thirst, but drinking the smallest amount makes the pain in the bladder worse, and it is vomited.

❖ **Burns**
Second- and third-degree burns and scalds.

WOMEN

❖ **Pruritis vulvae**
Burning and itching of vulva and vagina.

MEN

❖ **Genitals**
Painful swelling of genitals, with characteristic symptoms of *Cantharis*.

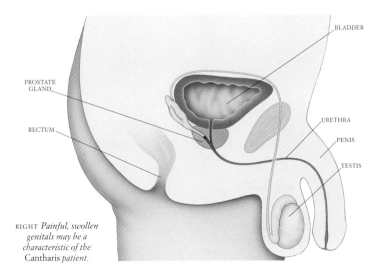

BLADDER

PROSTATE GLAND

RECTUM

URETHRA

PENIS

TESTIS

RIGHT *Painful, swollen genitals may be a characteristic of the* Cantharis *patient.*

Carbo vegetabilis

[CARB-V.]

Carbo vegetabilis *is derived from charcoal
from beech, poplar, or silver birch wood. In
homeopathy is it used as a remedy for restoring
vitality, and for flatulence. It is also thought to
have disinfectant and deodorizing properties.*

CONFIRMATION

Plant: CHARCOAL *wood or vegetable charcoal*

SENSATION
chilly

WORSE
warmth

BETTER
being fanned

- *Picture of collapse, with blue discoloration of skin*
- *Chilly, but wants to be fanned*
- *Burned out – low level of energy*
- *Accumulation of wind; offensive odors*

General indications
This remedy is known as the "corpse reviver" because it acts when there is a state of collapse or exhaustion, when the vitality is low. In the extreme condition, the person is pale, bluish, faint, cold, and weak, covered with cold sweat, and craves fresh air. Even the breath is cold. Though chilly, the person wants to be fanned. Digestion is weak and sluggish; there is flatulence with a foul odor. Useful for weaker children who do not fully recover from childhood diseases such as measles or whooping cough. Other less serious conditions can also benefit from this remedy.

Mental and emotional state
With the physical collapse, the mind is also weak. The person may be easily frightened, have memory loss, and seem not to care what happens.

Modalities
Worse: warmth; loss of vital fluids; cooling off. Better: burping; cool air and fanning.

Food/drink
Desires: salty foods. Aversions: fats, rich food.

RIGHT Carbo vegetabilis *is derived from charcoal and was first proved by Hahnemann himself.*

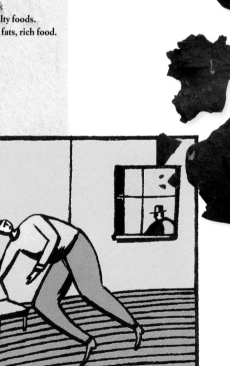

LEFT *The mental picture of* Carb-v. *may be of someone weak and easily startled.*

COMPLAINTS

❖ Common cold
Frequent and difficult sneezing, with a blocked nose. Tickle in the throat excites the sneeze, which aggravates the tickle.

❖ Cough
Hollow, choking cough, with headache and vomiting. Breathing is difficult, quick, and short. Chest feels as if it is burning, and this is made worse from drinking cold drinks. Whooping cough with blue face; cannot get enough air. Phlegm is thick, sticky, yellow, profuse.

❖ Fever
Alternate chill and heat. Icy coldness; warm head and cold limbs; internal burning heat with cold, icy skin and cold sweat.

❖ Digestive disorders
Digestion is slow. The abdomen is extremely bloated and distended with wind; the person cannot bear tight clothes around waist. Loud, sour belches temporarily relieves; much relief from passing wind. Indigestion from overeating, or from too-rich food.

❖ Symptoms of food poisoning
Painful diarrhea. Burning in rectum. Stool is putrid. Even soft stool is passed with difficulty.

CHILDREN

❖ Measles
With characteristic general, mental, fever, and other symptoms as applicable; mumps that progress to testicles or breast.

❖ Whooping cough
With characteristic *Carb-v.* general, mental, fever symptoms.

❖ Newborns
Give mother or baby a single dose crushed tablet (see Special Applications).

WOMEN

❖ Breastfeeding
Exhaustion after breastfeeding.

SPECIAL APPLICATIONS
Emergency first aid: newborn infant after long labor. Exhausted, cold, bluish. Carbon monoxide poisoning; exposure to car exhaust fumes causing sleepiness, weakness, exhaustion. Collapse of the elderly, with cold body, blue lips, weak pulse; demands open windows and fanning.

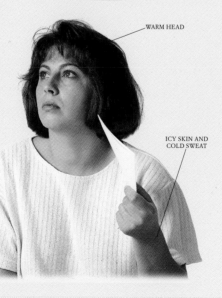

WARM HEAD

ICY SKIN AND COLD SWEAT

COLD LIMBS

RIGHT Carb-v. *patients are exhausted, cold and sweaty, but need to be fanned.*

COMPARISON OF REMEDIES
GENERAL

ARG-N.
Weakness and nervousness from anticipation of an ordeal. Warm blooded with craving for fresh air. Flatulence with loud explosive passing of wind.

CHINA
Weakness from loss of fluids. Oversensitive, nervous; marked periodicity. Restlessness of the affected parts. Worse for touch.

LYC.
Sore, pressing pain in liver on breathing, worse for touch. Constipation. Diarrhea from cold drinks.

VERAT.
Weakness, sudden collapse, chilliness, prostration, but intense thirst and profuse cold sweat. Copious diarrhea like rice-water, may be simultaneous with vomiting. Hands and feet are icy cold.

Caulophyllum

[CAUL.]

The Native Americans used Caulophyllum *as a herbal remedy to ease childbirth. The homeopathic tincture is made from the knotty root, gathered at the time of new growth. It is used homeopathically for labor that does not progress or for false labor pains.*

CONFIRMATION

Plant: CAULOPHYLLUM THALICTROIDES *papoose root, squaw root, blue cohosh*

WORSE
movement

BETTER
warmth

- *During childbirth, when labor is not progressing*
- *False labor pains*
- *Weakness during labor*

General indications
Mainly used during pregnancy. The uterus does not function properly. Cramps are low in the pelvis but the upper parts remain soft. Excessive weakness and nervous excitability during childbirth. False labor pains, labor that doesn't progress; unbearable afterpains. Pains are erratic, drawing, cramping, shooting, sharp, spasmodic.

Modalities
Worse: pregnancy; open air; coffee; motion. Better: warmth.

Food/drink
No marked desires or aversions.

RIGHT *The papoose root grows in North America.*

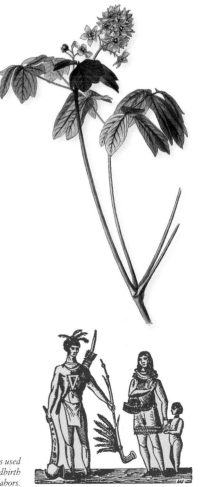

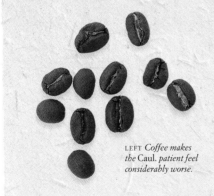

LEFT *Coffee makes the* Caul. *patient feel considerably worse.*

RIGHT *Native Americans used* Caulophyllum *during childbirth to relieve painful labors.*

COMPLAINTS

WOMEN

❖ **Labor pains**
In the first stage of labor, pains are ineffectual or irregular, or stop altogether; the cervix remains undilated.

❖ **Contractions**
May be weak, irregular, or strong, but in the lower abdomen. Pains fly in all directions, across the abdomen, into the groin, or down thighs.

❖ **Exhaustion from contractions**
With internal trembling. If this pattern remains after childbirth, *Caul.* can also be used for afterpains.

RIGHT *The remedy* Caulophyllum *is used to aid the progress of childbirth once labor has begun.*

CAUTION

Every remedy can also cause what it can cure; this is the basis of homeopathy. Therefore, *Caulophyllum* taken too early in pregnancy has the power to cause premature contractions.

COMPARISON OF REMEDIES
FOR CHILDBIRTH

ACON.
Shock after childbirth, or strong fear, especially of death, before childbirth.

ARN.
Soreness, bruised feelings and/or exhaustion after long, difficult labor. Any form of physical trauma or overexertion.

BELL-P.
Trauma of deep tissues, pelvic organs. After cesarian births when uterus becomes infected. General sensitivity to cold of any kind, or becoming suddenly cold.

CHAM.
Irregular labor pains traveling down the thighs. Extreme intolerable and distressing pain, with a desperate feeling. The person may shout, scream, or abuse others around.

CIMIC.
In labor, similar pains to *Caul.* but more violent, when cervix fails to dilate. The mood is distinctly gloomy, negative, or pessimistic, and the person feels unable to continue.

GELS.
False labor pains. Fear before childbirth with nervous diarrhea. This sort of fear has the effect of making the person sluggish, listless, drowsy – a sort of paralysis.

HYP.
Damage to nerves or nerve-rich tissues, therefore useful for pain after forceps delivery, cesarian incisions, episiotomy or epidural (after *Arn.*).

IP.
Nauseous symptoms predominate during labor.

PULS.
Labor pains that are not strong enough, irregular, ineffectual, or changing. Feeling overheated and worse in a stuffy room, and wanting the doors and windows open for fresh air. Feels emotionally sensitive, weepy, wants company and is better for gentle reassurance and affection.

SEP.
Dragging pains in the uterus. Pelvic floor or abdominal muscles are too relaxed. The person usually is much better for vigorous exercise. More useful after labor for postnatal trauma, muscles of pelvic floor remain too lax.

STAPH.
Pelvic pains after operation to sexual organs; episiotomy, cesarian section, abortion. The person may have strong feelings of anger, or of being emotionally injured from the experience as well, but feels unable to express them.

Causticum

[CAUST.]

Causticum is a remedy particular to homeopathy. It is made with a special preparation of lime and bisulfate of potash, using a process devised by Hahnemann in the early 19th century. It is used to treat severe burns, paralysis, and incontinence.

CONFIRMATION

Mineral: CAUSTICUM HAHNEMANNI *compound comprising* KALI *(potassium), calcium, and sulfur salts.*

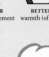

BETTER
gentle movement

BETTER
warmth (of bed)

THIRST
cold drinks

WORSE
open air

- *Burning pains, as if raw, sore, or open*
- *Better for sips of cold water*
- *Neuralgia, local paralysis*
- *Complaints feel better in damp weather*

General indications

Called for in cases of very serious burns (give while waiting for medical attention). Also for local paralytic affections, especially right-sided. Burning pains, like raw flesh of an open wound. Raw, sore pains. Wants to sip at cold water. Stammering from excitement or anger. Sensitive to authority; can't stand to see injustice. Neuralgic affections. Involuntary passing of urine on coughing or sneezing.

Mental and emotional state

Intensely sympathetic. Thinking of complaints makes the person feel worse. Melancholy mood, sadness, alternating with anxious, irritable, or hysterical mood. Looks on the dark side of life.

Modalities

Worse: dry, cold, or raw air; winds, drafts; evening, or 3–4 a.m.; clear fine weather.
Better: cold drinks (even during chill); damp wet weather; warmth of bed; gentle motion.

Food/drink

Desires: smoked meat and other foods, beer, cold drinks. Refreshing things, salty foods.
Aversions: candies.

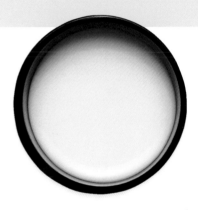

ABOVE *Lime and potassium bisulfate is the source for the* Causticum *remedy.*

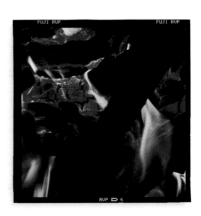

RIGHT Causticum *may be given as an emergency first aid treatment in the case of severe burns until medical help arrives.*

COMPLAINTS

❖ Eye complaints
Vision impaired, as if film before the eyes. Profuse acrid tears. Paralysis of eyes after exposure to cold. Dryness, photophobia. Pressure, as if from sand, in the eyes.

❖ Sore throat, laryngitis
Burning and rawness in the throat, with constant desire to swallow. Choking sensation. Difficulty in swallowing, or unable to hawk out mucus. Scraping down back of throat, with dryness. Laryngitis (especially in singers). Hoarseness persists after sore throat is better.

❖ Cough
Hollow, hard, dry cough, with rawness and soreness of chest; better for drinking cold water. Cannot cough deep enough to expel phlegm or mucus – must swallow it again. Dry, tickling cough, worse in cold air. Cough with pain in the hips.

❖ Incontinence, urine retention
Involuntary urination when coughing or sneezing, walking, or blowing the nose. Retention of urine: after surgical operations; after labor.

❖ Cystitis
Constant urge to urinate, but difficulty in actually passing. Burning in urethra when urinating; pain in the bladder after passing a few drops.

❖ Burns
Third-degree burns, scalds, or chemical burns. Burning pain, with blisters. Ill effects from burns; old burns that do not get well.

MEN

❖ Prostate
Enlarged, inflamed. Bruised soreness in testes.

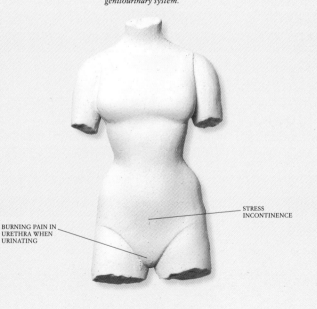

BELOW Causticum *is an important remedy for the genitourinary system.*

BURNING PAIN IN URETHRA WHEN URINATING

STRESS INCONTINENCE

COMPARISON OF REMEDIES

GENERAL

CAL.
For use in the later stages of healing of second- or third-degree burns, after blisters have burst. Helps prevent pus formation and promotes healthy new growth of skin. Soothes sunburn and rashes, heals raw and cracked area.

CANTH.
Second-degree burns with violent pains. Burns before blisters form. Burns with rawness and smarting.

URT-U.
First-degree burns, also urticaria, nettle rash. Worse after bathing or violent exercise. Violent itching. Burn confined to skin. Burning, stinging pains.

PHOS.
Hard, dry, tight cough, which may be violent, exhausting, or cause trembling. Coughs up a lot of phlegm. With the cough there is a burning sensation in the air passages. Desires cold, iced drinks.

61

Chamomilla

[CHAM.]

Worshiped by the ancient Egyptians for its healing properties, the chamomile plant has been used in medicine for hundreds of years. It is a useful, calming remedy especially for children with difficulties during teething. The homeopathic tincture is prepared with the whole fresh flowering plant.

CONFIRMATION

Plant: MATRICARIA RECUTITA *German or wild chamomile*

SENSITIVE
oversensitive

WORSE
touch

WORSE
coffee/alcohol

THIRST
cold drinks

- *Excessive irritability; extreme sensitivity to outside influences*
- *Screams and shrieks with pain*
- *Child wants to be carried; contrary*
- *Foul temper. Asks for things and throws them away*
- *Teething babies*
- *Childbirth*
- *Mild disposition contra-indicates remedy*

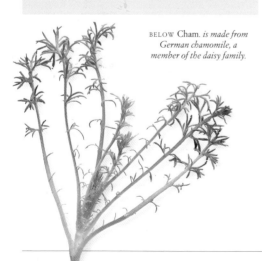

BELOW Cham. *is made from German chamomile, a member of the daisy family.*

General indications

Physical symptoms present with an extremely temperamental emotional state. Irritable. The person is in intolerable pain, mad with the pain. Whenever there is extreme sensitivity to pain, and an oversensitive mental state with it. Screams/shrieks with pain.

MOODY AND ILL-TEMPERED

RESPONSES ARE SNAPPY AND ABRUPT

Mental and emotional state

There is a vivid characteristic picture, which is always present with physical complaints. The person is highly emotional, temperamental, or oversensitive. Mood ugly, angry, quarrelsome, irritated by the smallest incident. Responses are snappy, abrupt. Child wants to be carried, demands many things but refuses them when given. Mild disposition rules out this remedy.

Modalities

Worse: coffee, alcohol; cold; touch.
Better: children are much better for being carried.

Food/drink

Desires: sour drinks. Aversions: coffee. Thirst: for cold drinks.

PERSON IS AGGRESSIVE AND UNPLEASANT

LEFT *The* Chamomilla *mood is irritable, aggressive, and ready for a fight.*

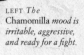

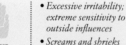

COMPLAINTS

❖ Earache
Extreme pain, relieved by warmth. Sensitive to cold wind, and noise; cannot stand music.

❖ Toothache
After warm drinks, in pregnancy.

❖ Cough
Dry, tickly cough; asthma attack from anger. Cough worse 9–12 p.m.

❖ Digestive disorders
Colic: pains after anger; sharp pain of wind. Worse at night; better for warm applications. Cheek becomes red with hot sweat. Indigestion; wind with odor of bad eggs. Bitter vomiting with bile; violent retching before vomiting.

❖ Diarrhea
Hot, sour, grass green, slimy; smelling of rotten eggs.

❖ Fever
Coldness of one part, heat of another: alternate chill and heat. Sweat on head; thirst during fever. Whole body cold, but face is burning hot. Foul-smelling sweat on head during sleep.

❖ Insomnia
Sleeplessness from anger, pain, or the use of stimulants, such as coffee.

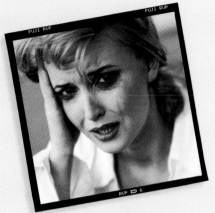

ABOVE Chamomilla *is indicated when the person is highly emotional and oversensitive.*

❖ Skin rash
Rash in infants and nursing mothers. Measles, with characteristic general, mental/emotional picture.

CHILDREN

❖ Teething pain
In babies, with one cheek hot or swollen, the other cold and pale. Green diarrhea.

❖ Hyperactivity
Chamomilla is best used in babies and young children. The child is overstimulated, irritable, restless, angry, quarrelsome, difficult to please. The remedy can help to calm the child in an acute instance of a tantrum, if given according to the *Chamomilla* state; also consult a professional homeopath.

❖ Measles
With characteristic *Chamomilla* general, mental, and fever symptoms.

WOMEN

❖ Childbirth
Labor pains are irregular, going down inner thighs. Intolerable pains with foul temper; she sends everyone away, screams, abuses those around her.

❖ Breastfeeding
Breast sore, nipples inflamed and tender; cramps when child nurses.

COMPARISON OF REMEDIES

GENERAL

COLOC.
Anger leading to physical complaints, especially cramps. Colic is better for bending double.

DIOS.
Child arches back and stretches limbs with severe pain in colic.

MAG-P.
Limbs drawn up with abdominal pain in colic. Better for hard pressure.

NUX V.
Irritable, but doesn't want to be touched. Complaints from overstimulation; indigestion with nausea.

PODO.
Noisy, spluttering, gushing stool. Diarrhea from teething.

China

[CHINA]

Derived from the Peruvian bark tree, China *was the first remedy that Hahnemann proved. The tincture is made from the stripped and dried bark of the tree. It is used to treat cases of nervous exhaustion and debility resulting from loss of bodily fluids or breastfeeding.*

General indications
Weakness and debility due to profuse, exhausting discharges – hemorrhages, diarrhea, suppuration, breastfeeding. The person is weak, oversensitive, nervous, anemic. Fevers tend to follow a pattern of periodicity – getting better and worse at regular intervals. Everything upsets – light, noise, odors. Pains are bursting. Profuse hemorrhages, with faintness, loss of sight, ringing in ears. Affects the digestive system. Face appears earthy, sickly, bluish around eyes. Extreme sensitivity to touch.

Mental and emotional state
Taciturn, ill-humored, hurts others' feelings, apathetic.

Modalities
Worse: touch; jarring; noise; cold winds; fruit, spoiled food, milk.
Better: hard pressure; loose clothes; warmth.

Food/drink
Desires: cold drinks, delicacies, spicy, highly seasoned foods, candies. Aversions: hot food, fats and rich food, fruit, meat, coffee, milk, beer.

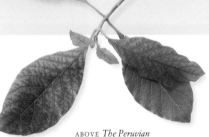

ABOVE *The Peruvian bark tree provides the source for* China, *the first homeopathic remedy.*

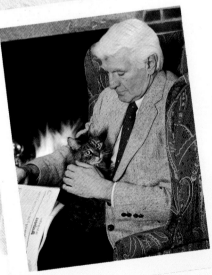

RIGHT *A desire for warmth is part of the* China *symptom picture.*

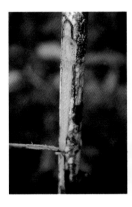

ABOVE *To make the* China *tincture, bark from the Peruvian bark tree is stripped and dried.*

COMPLAINTS

❖ Headache
Bursting throbbing pain; sensation that brain is loose in the head. Stitching pain from one side of the head to the other, after loss of fluids. Very sensitive to drafts and touch; better for hard pressure, rubbing. Extremely sensitive scalp. Face is earthy, sickly, bluish around eyes.

❖ Digestive disorders
Everything tastes bitter or salty. Easily satisfied when eating; aversion to all food. Loud belching that relieves; milk causes indigestion. Slow digestion; feels as if there is a weight in the stomach after eating a small quantity of food. Colic: relieved by bending double; hard pressure. Flatulent bloating, better for moving around; not better for passing wind. Fermentation in abdomen brought on by eating fruit.

BELOW China *may be needed when fruit causes colic or diarrhea.*

❖ Diarrhea
Undigested, brown, yellow, watery stool; bloody, painless. Diarrhea from fruit, milk, beer.

❖ Joint pain
Pains in limbs and joints as if sprained; feels worse for slight touch, but better for hard pressure.

❖ Skin sensitivity, rash
Extremely sensitive to touch. Measles.

❖ Fever
Stages are marked: chill, heat, and sweat; chill, then thirst, then heat, then thirst; red hot face, cold hands; drenching sweats at night; worse from the least motion, from weakness, from draining body fluids.

CHILDREN
❖ Measles
With characteristic *China* general, mental, and fever symptoms.

WOMEN
❖ Childbirth
Weakness from loss of blood during or after labor. Feels faint, chilly, hypersensitive to touch and noise.

SPECIAL APPLICATIONS
Postoperatively: After surgery the patient may experience weakness and faintness from blood loss. This feeling may last a long time after the operation. *China* can help rectify this. Also helps after abdominal surgery, when there is pain with distension of abdomen (other remedies are more distended than painful).

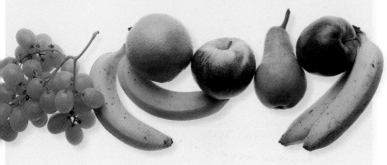

COMPARISON OF REMEDIES
FOR DEBILITY

CARB-V.
Complete prostration, wants to be fanned; better for open air.

LYC.
Sore pressing pain in liver, on breathing; worse for touch. Constipation: stool hard, difficult, small. Diarrhea from cold drinks. Sensitive, fearful, nervous before ordeals.

VERAT.
Another picture of weakness and sudden collapse. With *Verat.*, there is also intense thirst, and a profuse cold sweat. Diarrhea may be simultaneous with vomiting as if the whole body is trying to purge itself. Diarrhea is watery and copious, and can be forcefully evacuated, or almost involuntary; sweating before and after stool produces exhaustion. There may be cramping in muscles accompanying diarrhea; hands and feet remain icy cold. Suitable for gastroenteritis when the symptoms fit the picture.

Cimicifuga

[CIMIC.]

Cimicifuga *comes from a herb native to North America. The Native Americans used it as an antidote to snake bites, hence its common name of black snake-root. The homeopathic tincture is made from the root, which is crushed, steeped in alcohol, and strained.*

General indications
For problems with pregnancy, labor, and after childbirth. Depressed emotions accompany or alternate with physical symptoms. Pains are shooting, or shocklike, irregular, and shift quickly across the abdomen. Chilly, sensitive.

Mental and emotional state
Low spirited, depressed, gloomy, pessimistic, as if living in a black cloud where all is dark and confusing. **At other times talkative, excited, quickly changing subjects. Person thinks she is going crazy. Sighing is prominent.**

Modalities
Worse: cold, damp weather; drafts.
Better: wrapping warmly; gentle continued motion.

Food/drink
No marked desires or aversions.

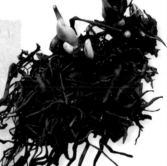

ABOVE *The* Cimicifuga *remedy is made from the fresh black snake-root.*

BELOW *The mental picture for* Cimicifuga *is gloomy and pessimistic.*

COMPLAINTS

WOMEN

❖ **Pregnancy**
Nausea in the morning; pain in lower back, through hips, and down thighs. Other complaints, with characteristic mental/ general symptoms.

❖ **Childbirth**
Pains move quickly from side to side across pelvis, instead of forcing downward. Contractions cease altogether, or are weak. Severe afterpains, sensitivity, intolerance to pain.

COMPARISON OF REMEDIES

LABOR PAINS

CAUL.
Exhaustion from contractions, which are irregular and/or ineffectual. Cervix remains undilated. Contractions in the lower abdomen, with softness at the top of the uterus.

SEP.
Severe bearing-down pains; dragging in uterus; dislikes fuss and sympathy.

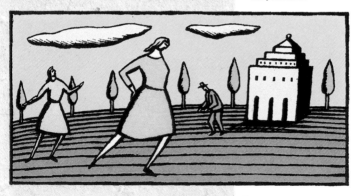

Cocculus indicus

[COCC.]

Also known as the Indian cockle, Cocculus
indicus *comes from the fruits of the* Anamirta
cocculus *species. Seeds are ground to a powder to
prepare the tincture. It is the main homeopathic
remedy for travel sickness, and is also used to
treat morning sickness during pregnancy.*

General indications
**This remedy is often used
for nausea and dizziness.
Sea sickness, or motion
sickness, and nausea
during pregnancy.
Feeling faint. Unusually,
the person is worse in
the fresh air.**

Mental and
emotional state
**Excited, or weak
and confused.**

Modalities
**Worse: fresh air; after
eating and drinking;
movement, sitting up.
Better: lying down – the
person must lie down to
prevent vomiting.**

Food/drink
**Desires: cold drinks, beer.
Aversions: food, the smell
of food (but may be
hungry at the same time).**

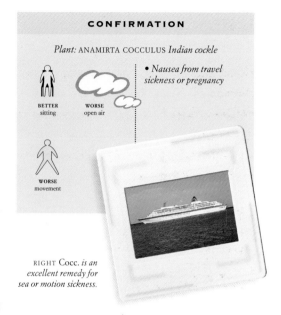

CONFIRMATION

Plant: ANAMIRTA COCCULUS *Indian cockle*

BETTER
sitting

WORSE
open air

• *Nausea from travel
sickness or pregnancy*

WORSE
movement

RIGHT Cocc. *is an
excellent remedy for
sea or motion sickness.*

COMPARISON OF REMEDIES

NAUSEA

ARS.
Nausea, vomiting, and
diarrhea as from food
poisoning. Restlessness.
Thirst for cold drinks that
are drunk in sips.

IGN.
Nausea, empty sensation in
the stomach that feels better
after eating. Symptoms arise
from intense emotional
grief, or love
disappointment.

IP.
Nausea symptoms
predominate, with
thirstlessness. Less dizziness
and vertigo than *Cocc.*

NUX V.
Irritability. Nausea from
overindulgence in food and
drink. Desire to vomit but
cannot.

SEP.
Nausea in pregnancy before
eating; vomiting food and bile
in the morning. Generally
worse for hormonal changes.

COMPLAINTS

❖ **Travel sickness**
Caused or made worse
from watching the
movement of
surroundings (i.e. looking
out of the window while
riding in a car, or
watching other boats or
movement at sea, etc.).
Headache, dizziness,
nausea, feeling faint.

❖ **Nausea**
At the thought of, or smell
of, food, or just looking at
food. Nervousness and
weakness generally.
The person may be
experiencing a
combination of physical
and emotional stress.

WOMEN

❖ **Pregnancy**
Nausea.

LEFT *The Indian
cockle is the source for
Cocculus indicus.*

67

Colocynthis

[COLOC.]

Colocynthis *was used as a purgative by Greek and Arab physicians. The remedy comes from a bitter and poisonous gourd known as bitter cucumber. The dried fruit is powdered, steeped in alcohol, then strained to make the tincture. It is used to treat cramps and colic.*

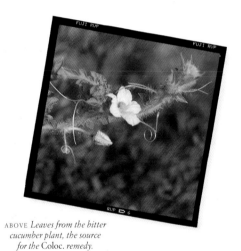

ABOVE *Leaves from the bitter cucumber plant, the source for the* Coloc. *remedy.*

General indications and complaints
This remedy is used mainly for abdominal cramps. Pains are sudden and violent; cramping, cutting, gnawing. Colic that comes on after overexcitement, anger, or indigestion. May be the effects of eating unripe or rotten fruit, or drinking bad water (unclean water in a tropical country). The pain is better when bending over double or pressing hard on the abdomen. With nausea, vomiting, diarrhea. Babies with colic prefer being held over the shoulder, which provides pressure to the abdomen.

CONFIRMATION

Plant: COLOCYNTHIS VULGARIS *bitter cucumber*

ONSET
sudden

BETTER
pressure

WORSE
overexcitement

- *Colic, abdominal cramps after overexcitement, anger or eating unripe or rotten fruit*
- *Sudden violent pain, better when bending double or pressing hard on abdomen*
- *Colic in babies*

COMPARISON OF REMEDIES

FOR COLIC

DIOS.
Colic in babies who arch their backs and extend their legs with the pain. They feel worse when doubled up, so prefer to be held upright.

MAG-P.
Spasms, cramps in stomach. Pain is not relieved by belching. Feels as if there is a tight band around the body. Colic due to flatulence. Cramping pain that is relieved by bending double, warmth, and pressure. Limbs are drawn up with pain during colic.

NUX V.
Colic, indigestion from overeating with nausea. There is a sensation of weight in the stomach, which is sensitive to pressure. Wants to vomit but cannot.

STAPH.
Colic and indigestion caused by anger with feelings of being emotional and/or physically insulted or injured.

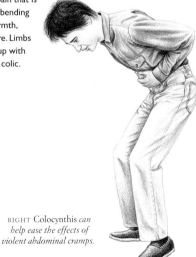

RIGHT Colocynthis *can help ease the effects of violent abdominal cramps.*

Dioscorea

[DIOS.]

A native of the United States, the wild yam is used homeopathically to treat colic in babies. To prepare the remedy, the root is macerated and steeped in alcohol and the mixture is then strained to prepare the tincture. The plant was used in the first female oral contraceptives and is also used as a natural source of progesterone.

CONFIRMATION

Plant: DIOSCOREA VILLOSA *colic root, wild yam*

BETTER
upright

WORSE
early morning
−2 a.m. onward

- *Colic in babies*
- *Better for bending backward or stretching out*

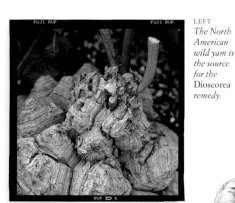

LEFT *The North American wild yam is the source for the Dioscorea remedy.*

General indications
This remedy has a particular use for unbearable, griping colic, which is worse for doubling up and is relieved by stretching out or bending backward. Babies with colic arch their backs and extend their legs; they feel better when held upright, and they do not want to lie down.

Modalities
Better: being held upright.
Worse: lying down.

COMPARISON OF REMEDIES

COLIC

ARS.
Violent abdominal pains cause extreme anguish and restlessness because the person cannot get comfortable. Burning pains are relieved by heat. These pains accompany symptoms of food poisoning with nausea, vomiting, and diarrhea.

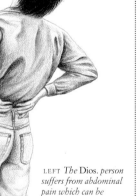

LEFT *The* Dios. *person suffers from abdominal pain which can be relieved by bending backward.*

Thirst for cold water, which is drunk in sips; or, craves ice water, which is vomited immediately after drinking.

COLOC.
Colic relieved by bending double or drawing the knees up, and by pressing hard on the abdomen. Babies with colic prefer to be held over the shoulder.

IP.
Colic pains are worse from moving around. Complaints usually include nausea, where the person wants to vomit, but vomiting does not relieve the nausea (in *Nux-v.*, vomiting does relieve). Frequent diarrhea of green slimy stool. Stomach pains may follow an experience of extreme anger.

PULS.
Pains in the lower abdomen shift around and cause rumbling, gurgling noises. Stomach aches are caused by fatty, rich food. The person is generally mild tempered, wanting company and affection, to the point of clinging. Warm blooded, better in the open cool air.

Drosera

[DROS.]

This insectivorous plant is found throughout the world in damp, boggy conditions. In the Middle Ages it was used as a remedy for the plague. The whole fresh plant, picked when in flower, is used to make the homeopathic tincture. It is used to treat coughs, sore throats, and fevers.

CONFIRMATION

Plant: DROSERA ROTUNDIFLORA *roundleaved sundew*

WORSE
midnight

WORSE
warmth

BETTER
open air

- *Preeminently a cough remedy, especially whooping cough*
- *Restless*
- *Paroxysmal, spasmodic cough, with retching, vomiting, nosebleed, and cold sweat*
- *Worse for warmth; better for open air*

General indications
The respiratory organs are primarily affected, with spasm, catarrh, hemorrhages; tight, constrictive pains in the throat, larynx, and stomach. History of tuberculosis in the family.

personally; imagines being deceived, persecuted. Restless, with poor concentration.

Modalities
**Worse: midnight; lying down; warmth.
Better: pressure; open air.**

Mental and
emotional state
Mistrustful, easily angered. Takes things

Food/drink
No marked desires or aversions.

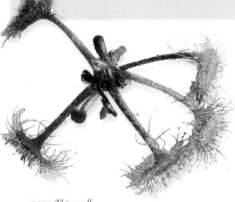

ABOVE *This small carnivorous sundew plant is the source for* Drosera.

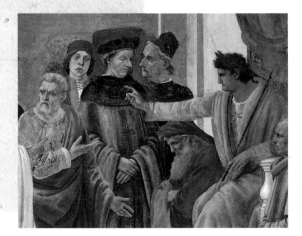

LEFT *A* Drosera *state is characterized by a deep sense of persecution.*

COMPLAINTS

❖ **Nosebleed**
With whooping cough.

❖ **Sore throat, laryngitis**
Tickling sensation as if
there is a feather in the
throat. Swallowing
solid food is difficult.
Dryness causes a
hacking cough with
hoarse, deep voice.
Yellow and green
mucus comes up
from throat.

❖ **Cough**
Chest feels tight,
constricted. Tickling in
larynx causes cough.
Fits of rapid, deep
barking or choking
cough; prolonged
incessant cough. Cough
seems to come from
the abdomen, and takes
the breath away. The
person is compelled to
hold the sides.
Followed by retching
and vomiting. Voice
deep, hoarse, or hollow,
and toneless. Whooping
cough. Difficulty
breathing out.

❖ **Aches and pains**
Limbs feel sore; bed
feels hard; pain in
long bones.

❖ **Fever**
Always too cold;
fever with
whooping cough.
Face becomes
hot; hands
become cold
with shivering.

COMPARISON OF REMEDIES
FOR COUGH

ANT-T.
Chest is full of mucus, the
person is too weak to cough
it up. Sleepy, drowsy, too
relaxed, lacking in reaction.
Shallow breathing from
inability to clear chest; worse
in a warm room, better for
expectoration and sitting up.

BELOW Drosera *is one
of the main remedies
to consider taking
for chest complaints.*

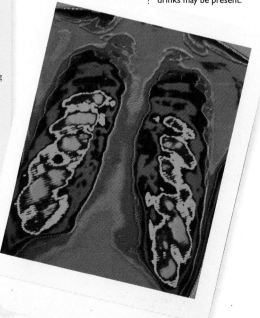

BELL.
Rapid and vigorous onset of
complaints. Cough is short,
dry, barking. Child feels a pain
in the stomach before an
attack of whooping cough,
and cries before the cough.
Larynx is very painful, the
throat is dry and hot. The
Bell. picture is of a face that
is fiery red and hot, or
alternately pale and red;
pupils of eyes dilated; pains
throbbing, sharp, or shooting.
Violent mental states or
hallucinations often
accompany physical symptoms.
No thirst during a fever, but a
desire for lemons or lemon
drinks may be present.

CARB-V.
A state of collapse or
exhaustion with low vitality
and cold sweat. Slow onset
of symptoms. Breathing is
difficult, quick, and short,
with a burning feeling in the
chest. This is made worse
from drinking cold drinks.
Hollow, choking cough, with
headache and vomiting. The
person cannot get enough
air, becomes blue in the face,
and must be fanned. The
beginning stages of whooping
cough, when no other
remedy is clearly indicated.

IP.
Cough with continuous
nausea, or cough causes
vomiting without nausea.
Constant and violent cough.
The child stiffens out with
the cough, becomes
nauseous, then vomits. Dry,
spasmodic cough ending in
choking or gagging.
Whooping cough with
nosebleed. Children difficult
to please. Constriction in the
chest feels worse from
movement. The chest is full
of phlegm, with loose coarse
rattling, but no phlegm is
brought up (similar to *Ant-t.,*
but less weak). These
symptoms are worse from
cold air, but better from cold
drinks and warmth.

Euphrasia
[EUPH.]

As its common name of eyebright suggests, Euphrasia is used primarily to treat conditions of the eye. It was first used in the 14th century by the herbalist Hildegarde. The expressed juice of the plant is mixed with alcohol to make the homeopathic tincture.

General indications
The *Euphrasia* remedy affects the eyes, particularly the mucous membranes. Burning acrid tears sting. Hayfever, conjunctivitis, colds, coughs, and other complaints that affect the eye in this way. Worse in the evening.

Mental and emotional state
No marked symptoms.

Modalities
Worse: sunlight, wind, warmth, smoke; after a long sleep; in the evening. Better: bathing the eyes.

Food/drink
No marked desires or aversions.

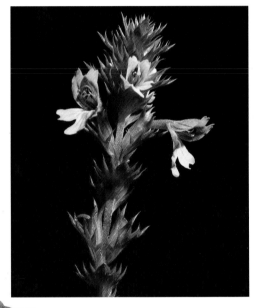

ABOVE *Eyebright is a semiparisitic wildflower that is always found with certain meadow grasses.*

LEFT *The* Euphrasia *picture is characterized by stinging, painful eyes that are relieved by bathing.*

COMPLAINTS

❖ **Eye complaints**
Burning, stinging, as if there is sand in the eyes. Acrid tears on coughing, in the wind, with cold in the nose, during a headache. Margins are raw, burning, swollen, and itching. Dilute tincture to use as eyebath for relief of sore eyes.

❖ **Hayfever**
Stinging eyes with bland nasal discharge. Sneezing.

❖ **Cough**
Forceful in the daytime. Better for lying down. Large quantities of mucus are brought up.

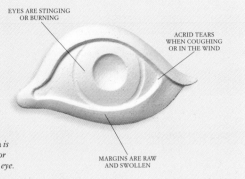

EYES ARE STINGING OR BURNING

ACRID TEARS WHEN COUGHING OR IN THE WIND

MARGINS ARE RAW AND SWOLLEN

RIGHT *Euphrasia is a useful remedy for complaints of the eye.*

COMPARISON OF REMEDIES
FOR THE EYE

ALL-C.
Eyes burn, lens discharge is watery, bland, and non-irritating. The nose produces a profuse watery, acrid, discharge that leaves sores on the nostrils and upper lip. Worse in a warm room or during cold weather and in the evening. Symptoms are better in the open air.

ARS.
Nose feels blocked, yet produces a thin, watery, fluent running discharge that causes soreness of the upper lip. General characteristics include chilliness, restlessness, and fussiness for details. Symptoms are worse after midnight, from 1–2 a.m.

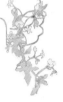

BRY.
Watery, achy eyes with headache, sneezing, and runny nose. Colds develop slowly. Headaches accompany most complaints. The most important characteristic is that the least movement or exertion makes the whole person or the complaint much worse.

GELS.
Colds, flu, inflammations that come on slowly. Eyes are red, sore, and aching. The general action of *Gels.* is on muscles, so eyes may be affected by dim or double vision.

The nose feels blocked and dry, though it may be runny with a watery, acrid discharge. The person generally feels drowsy, exhausted, listless, wants to lie and be still. Unlike *Bry.*, when the pain is worse from movement, *Gels.* lies motionless because of tiredness and weakness.

MERC.
Watery eyes with burning discharge. Inflammations with discharge of pus. Discharges are generally profuse, foul, and offensive. *Merc.* generally affects the glands with increased secretions such as saliva and sweat. The person may be much worse for heat or cold.

NAT-M.
Vision blurred, wavering. Pain when looking down. Tears stream down face with coughing. Worse in the morning.

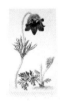

PULS.
Conjunctivitis with thick, yellow, bland discharge causing the eyelids to stick together. Sties of the upper eyelids that feel better with warm or cold bathing. The person is generally warm, and feels better in the open air. Suited to affectionate, wild emotional people who crave sympathy and attention.

Gelsemium

[GELS.]

Gelsemium is prepared from false or yellow jasmine, a climbing plant native to North America. To make the remedy, the root of the plant is chopped, steeped in alcohol, then strained to make the tincture. It is used to treat headaches, fevers, and may be given as a calming remedy.

CONFIRMATION

Plant: GELSEMIUM SEMPERVIRENS *yellow jasmine*

ONSET
slow

WORSE
heat of sun

THIRST
absent

- *Heavy, listless, drowsy in flu or cold*
- *Aching*
- *Slow onset*
- *No thirst*
- *Anticipating ordeals, feels paralyzed*

General indications
Gelsemium **acts primarily on the muscles, causing muscle aches, tiredness, weakness, and on the nerves, causing trembling, twitching, and paralysis. Emotions are affected by any sudden shock or surprise. The person feels exhausted, sluggish, heavy, drowsy, listless, wants to lie down, and is worse for movement. There may be dizziness. Arms and legs are weak and trembling.**
Gelsemium **is an excellent remedy for colds, flu, inflammations, childhood diseases, and anticipatory anxiety.**

Mental and emotional state
Dazed, apathetic, dull, listless, wants to be quiet, left alone, doesn't care about the illness, and so is worse from the stimulation of sudden emotions, shock. Dreads forthcoming ordeals.

Modalities
Worse: shocks (sudden news); oppressive, damp, humid weather; heat of sun in summer. Better: profuse urination, sweating.

Food/drink
No marked desires or aversions.
THIRST: **none during fever.**

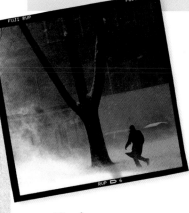

ABOVE *Misty, damp weather aggravates the symptoms of the* Gelsemium *mental state.*

LEFT *Yellow jasmine, the source for* Gelsemium, *is a climbing plant with fragrant flowers.*

COMPLAINTS

❖ Emotional problems

Anxiety from anticipation of an ordeal; nervous diarrhea before exams or any sort of test. Any situation in which there is fearful anticipation, such as before childbirth.

❖ Headache

Headache heavy, feeling like a band around the back of the head that spreads from the neck over the back of head to forehead and eyes. Head feels better from lying with the head raised. A peculiar symptom is that the headache is better after profuse urination.

❖ Eye complaints

Eyes red, sore, and aching; pupils dilated; sight dim; blurred or double vision.

❖ Common cold

Nose runny with a watery acrid discharge, even though it feels stuffed and dry. Feels as though hot water is coming out of the nose. Colds worse in the

summer. Sneezing particularly in the morning. Pain from throat to ear, feeling there is a lump in the throat that cannot be swallowed. Chest is sore with a dry cough.

❖ Influenza

Onset of symptoms is slow, a few days after exposure, often in the mild, damp, and humid weather of spring or fall. The person feels heavy and unable to move. Aches all over. Arms and legs are weak and trembly. Face is dusky red with a lack of expression. Tongue is covered with a thick, yellow coating. Eyelids droop, and it is difficult to open them. Fever accompanied by chills and dull pains up and down the spine, and cold sweat. Face is hot, though limbs are cold. Thirst is usually absent, but there may be thirst with sweating. Appetite is lacking, but the person will take some food and drink. Copious, watery, pale urine. An unusual, but

characteristic symptom is a feeling in the heart that the person must keep moving or else the heart will stop.

❖ Diarrhea

Yellow or green stool, painless.

❖ Skin eruptions

Hot, dry, itching eruptions on skin.

CHILDREN

❖ Measles

Gelsemium will help to bring out eruptions, and relieve general symptoms, with characteristic symptoms of the remedy.

WOMEN

❖ Pregnancy and Childbirth

Gelsemium affects muscles, nerves, and emotions, so it is good for false labor pains. Fear before childbirth; nervous diarrhea before childbirth. Threatened abortion from sudden depressing emotion. Nervous chills in first stages of labor.

COMPARISON OF REMEDIES

GENERAL

ACON.
Rapid onset; fearful; thirsty for cold drinks; ailments from cold dry winds, or fright.

BELL.
Rapid onset, red face/throat; hot body, cold hands/feet, right-sided; delusions/delirium.

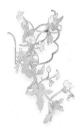

BRY.
Any movement causes pain, wants to stay completely still; thirsty for large quantities.

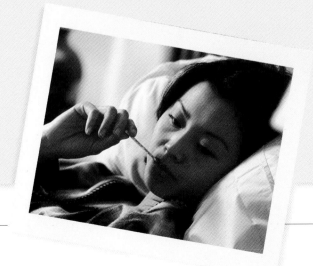

LEFT Gelsemium *is one of the key homeopathic remedies to take for influenza.*

Hamamelis

[HAM.]

The Hamamelis *remedy is prepared from the bark of the witch hazel tree. The fresh bark is macerated, steeped in alcohol, and the resulting mixture is then strained to make the tincture. The homeopathic remedy is used to treat hemorrhoids, varicose veins, and hemorrhages.*

CONFIRMATION

Tree: HAMAMELIS VIRGINIANA *witch hazel*

WORSE
open air

WORSE
touch/pressure

AVERSION
water

- *Hemorrhages from injuries*
- *Parts feel sore, bruised, painful*
- *Distended veins*
- *Bleeding hemorrhoids*

General indications
Hamamelis **should be taken internally for the complaints listed. However, a cream or ointment is also available, which can be applied to bruised and broken areas of skin. The remedy is used primarily for venous congestions, varicose veins, hemorrhoids, and hemorrhages. The parts affected feel bruised and sore.**

Mental and emotional state
No marked symptoms.

Modalities
Worse: pressure; open air; injuries.
Better: rest, lying quietly.

Food/drink
Aversion to water; thinking of water causes nausea.

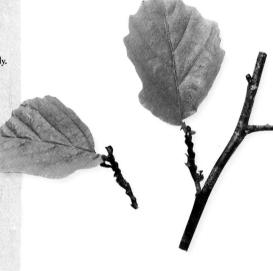

ABOVE *Bark is stripped from the twigs of the witch hazel tree to make the* Hamamelis *remedy.*

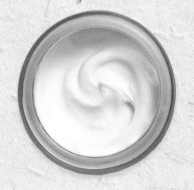

LEFT *The* Ham. *remedy is available as a cream and may be applied directly to bruised skin.*

COMPLAINTS

❖ **Black eye**
Bruising after injury to eye. Try *Arn.* first; if vision is affected try *Ham.*

❖ **Nosebleed**
With dark, thin blood, especially after a blow to the nose; continues for a long time.

❖ **Bleeding gums**
Excessive bleeding after tooth extraction.

❖ **Hemorrhages**
Affected part is sore, bruised, painful to the touch. Any bleeding from injuries, blows, etc.

WOMEN

❖ **Varicose veins**
During pregnancy: hard, swollen, and sensitive to touch.

❖ **Bleeding hemorrhoids**
In late pregnancy or after childbirth; may be exhausting even if only a small amount of blood is lost.

BELOW Hamamelis *is an excellent remedy for nosebleeds, particularly those that continue for a long time.*

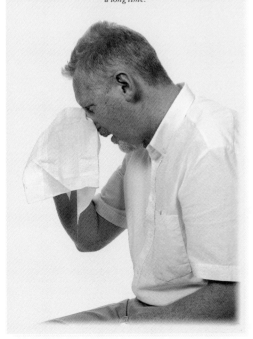

COMPARISON OF REMEDIES
FOR NOSEBLEEDS

CARB-V.
When nosebleeds occur in daily attacks, especially in the morning, then think of *Carb-v.* There is the characteristic pale tending to bluish color in the face (before and after each attack) though there may be a red tip on the end of the nose. Usually accompanies much sneezing (e.g. colds, hayfever, asthma) but the person feels much worse after sneezing. Recurrent nosebleeds, especially in those who are overanxious, especially the elderly. There may also be varicose veins on the nose.

DROS.
Nosebleeds of *Drosera* type are usually associated with whooping cough. *Drosera* being one of the main remedies for that disease. It therefore tends to come on from coughing, but may also occur after stooping. Sneezing may be very painful, and person is very sensitive to sour smells.

IP.
Also useful when nosebleed is associated with whooping cough, but the characteristic *Ip.* nausea would almost certainly be part of the picture. In a child, the nosebleed occurs from a constant and violent cough, ending in choking and gagging, or vomiting.

PHOS.
By contrast, blood from a *Phosphorus* nosebleed will have the *Phos.* general characteristics – blood is bright red. Although the nosebleeds occur quite easily, they are quite small hemorrhages. It may occur during the cough, or stool, in extremis instead of menses. The *Phos.* person with a nosebleed will also be oversensitive to smell, but especially during a headache.

PULS.
Pulsatilla also has an affinity with hormonally related problems, so nosebleeds may occur before and during menses, and from suppressed menses, and also with frequent sneezing. General characteristics of *Pulsatilla* still apply – person will feel better in the open air, and worse indoors in a stuffy atmosphere.

SUL.
Sulfur person, also dry and not thirsty like *Puls.*, may have easy bleeding, like other *Sulfur* symptoms, worse at night. Nosebleeds are accompanied by itching and burning in the nose, with violent, fluent coryza and frequent sneezing.

Hepar sulfuris calcareum
[HEP.]

Hep. is prepared from equal parts of powdered oystershells and pure flowers of sulfur. It is kept at white heat for ten minutes, dissolved in hydrocholic acid, then triturated. Hahnemann used it to treat the side effects of mercury, commonly used in 18th-century medicines.

CONFIRMATION

Mineral: CALCIUM SULFIDE

SENSATION
chilly

SENSITIVE
oversensitive

WORSE
touch

BETTER
heat

- Touchy, oversensitive to pain, cold, touch, noise, odors, outside influences
- Hates the cold or slightest draft; must be warmly wrapped
- Violent, intense pain
- Sour and smelly discharges

General indications
Great sensitivity to the slightest pain, cold, touch, noise, odors, flow of air. Onset and progress of the illness are sudden and rapid. Mucous membranes of the respiratory system are affected – ears, nose throat, lungs. With the inflammation are swollen glands and the formation of much thick pus. All discharges – pus, sweat, stool, etc. – are profuse and foul, smelling sour or cheesy. The person is very chilly, but sweats easily, and the sweat does not relieve. Pains are sore and very sharp, like splinters. Illness often comes on after exposure to cold and dry wind.

Mental and emotional state
Oversensitivity shows in touchiness. Irritable from the pain; dissatisfied with everything, quarrelsome, and may become violent with anger, and may express a desire to kill.

Modalities
Worse: Cold, dry air, drafts, uncovering, touch. Must not lie on the part that is painful. Worse for onset at night. **Better:** warm wrapping, moist heat, damp weather.

Food/drink
Desires: strong craving for vinegar, acidic drinks. **Aversions:** fatty food.

BELOW *A characteristic Hep. pain is sharp and feels like a fishbone caught in the throat.*

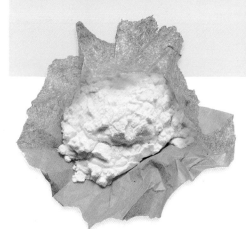

ABOVE *Flowers of sulfur, which are mixed with oystershell powder to make the remedy.*

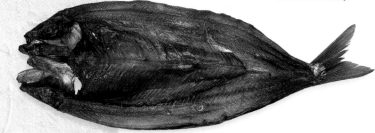

COMPLAINTS

❖ Headache
Headache boring into the right side, root of nose. Worse for movement, stooping. Headpain from exposure to dry cold or cold wind, or any draft.

❖ Tooth abscesses
With mental and/or general symptoms.

❖ Earache
Infection, with sharp, shooting pain. Discharge of foul-smelling pus from the ear. Child will cry out. The child may put a hand over the ear in order to keep it warm.

❖ Common cold
Nose may be runny, blocked, or sneezing, occurs after being in a cold wind. Sour or cheesy discharge. Best prescribed in the later stages of a cold, after *Aconite*.

❖ Sore throat
Swollen tonsils and neck glands. Pain as if a splinter is stuck in the throat; extends to the ears when yawning or swallowing. Laryngitis and hoarseness from being out in the cold wind. Warm drinks make the throat feel better.

❖ Cough
Cough is barking and choking; throat irritated, as if tickled by a feather. Worse from cold drinks or cold air. Cries from pain before coughing. Chest is weak; there is much rattling, and large amounts of loose, yellow phlegm that is brought up with difficulty.

❖ Skin eruptions
Ulcers, cold sores, and boils: inflamed and very sensitive to touch. Every injury to the skin is slow to heal, producing foul-smelling pus.

❖ Fevers
Low grade, but there is a great deal of sweat, which is sour and offensive.

HEADACHE ON RIGHT SIDE AND ROOT OF NOSE

HAS SLIGHT FEVER, WITH MUCH SWEATING

FEEL BETTER IF WRAPPED UP WARMLY

RIGHT Hep. *is a valuable remedy for coughs, colds, and flu.*

COMPARISON OF REMEDIES

GENERAL

MERC.
Swollen glands, increased secretions, profuse offensive discharges that are thin, acrid, and burning or thick yellow-green. Worse for becoming overheated as well as chilled; worse at night. Easy and profuse perspiration that does not relieve.

SIL.
Sensitive, thirsty, chilly, sweaty; every little injury to skin becomes infected. Timid, yielding nature, but with inner resistance.

Hypericum

[HYP.]

Hypericum, or St. John's wort, has long been used by herbalists as a wound remedy and also as a treatment for mild depression. In homeopathy, the whole flowering plant is chopped and steeped in alcohol to make the tincture.

General indications
First aid: any injury and damage to nerve-rich tissues, causing excruciating pain. Shooting pains with tingling or burning, or there may be numbness in the part.

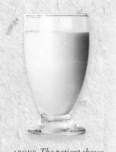

Mental and emotional state
No marked symptoms.

ABOVE *The patient shows a desire for hot milk when* Hypericum *is indicated.*

Modalities
Worse: touch; motion, being moved or jarred; cold air.
Better: lying quietly.

Food/drink
Desires: warm drinks, milk.
No marked aversions.

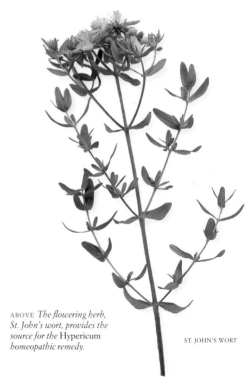

ABOVE *The flowering herb, St. John's wort, provides the source for the* Hypericum *homeopathic remedy.*

ST. JOHN'S WORT

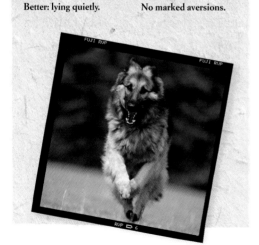

LEFT Hypericum *is often prescribed for puncture wounds, including dog bites.*

COMPLAINTS

❖ **Hair loss**
Hair falls out after head injury, concussion.

❖ **Toothache**
After dental care, when there is pain in teeth or jaw after anesthetic wears off. Shooting pains in the gums after tooth extraction.

❖ **Hemorrhoids**
With pain, bleeding, and soreness.

❖ **Injuries, wounds**
Especially good for ends of fingers or toes. For example, after hitting thumb with a hammer or crushing fingertips. Falling on spine or coccyx. Use before surgery on spine. Concussion. Animal bites. Wounds caused by nails or splinters; severe lacerations, scrapes, and grazes. Recovery from surgical incisions. Prevents tetanus after puncture wounds. Any effects resulting from injuries to the head or spine, such as headache, dizziness, continued pain in the coccyx.

❖ **Bed sores**
Apply external cream; take internally when there is sharp, shooting pain.

WOMEN

❖ **Childbirth**
Sharp, shooting pains continue after forceps delivery, epidural, episiotomy, cesarian.

> **SPECIAL APPLICATIONS**
> Use after surgical procedures with painful incisions; before surgery on spine. Continued pain in the location of an injection from a needle.

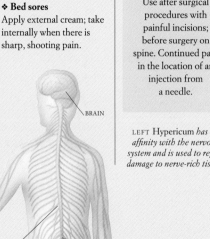

LEFT Hypericum *has an affinity with the nervous system and is used to repair damage to nerve-rich tissue.*

BRAIN

SPINAL NERVES OF THE PERIPHERAL NERVOUS SYSTEM

SPINAL CORD

SCIATIC NERVE

ARN.
The first remedy to consider in cases of trauma and injury where there is a sore, bruised feeling, or general physical shock such as with accidents, falls, broken bones, sprains or strains of joints, surgery, childbirth. Other remedies may be indicated after the initial phase of trauma has subsided. Reconsider the symptoms and the condition to determine which remedy is best suited to the picture that develops. *Arnica* cream can be applied as long as there is no broken skin.

LED.
Puncture wounds from sharp pointed instruments, needles, nails, knives, or animal and insect bites. The part affected becomes swollen and numb with a pale or mottled black-and-blue appearance, and is painful to touch. It feels cold externally, and the pain is relieved by the application of cold compresses or cold water. Sprained joints that are worse for any movement, feel cold to the touch, and are better for cold applications.

Ignatia amara

[IGN.]

Introduced to Europe from the Far East by Spanish Jesuits in the 17th century, Ignatia amara is used mainly for emotional upsets and problems. The bean is ground to a fine powder, steeped in alcohol, then strained to make the homeopathic tincture.

CONFIRMATION

Plant: STRYCHNOS IGNATII *St. Ignatius' bean*

WORSE touch

WORSE candy

WORSE smoke

BETTER eating

- *Acute emotional upset*
- *Complaints after emotional conflict*
- *Changeable, contradictory physical states*
- *Sighing*

General indications

The emotional state is usually foremost; it is often caused by grief or anxiety. The nervous system is affected with spasms or tremors. It is excellent for an immediate, acute state of grief, with irrational worries caused by feelings of great disappointment, loss, or jealousy. Because the emotions are disturbed, the person may change rapidly from one condition to its opposite – such as crying one moment, laughing the next. This tendency toward fluctuation or contradictory behavior appears on the physical level as well. Acute illnesses following deep emotional shock or loss, breakup of relationships, homesickness. Physical symptoms directly related to the overt or suppressed emotions.

Mental and emotional state

Brooding and moody, silent and sad, crying and sighing. Emotional upheaval causes instability and nervousness. Cause may be the death of a loved one, or a love disappointment; being reprimanded; or suppressing these emotions. The person might be angry, anguished, sobbing, laughing hysterically, intolerant, impatient, or introspective at different times. Prefers to be alone; does not like to be comforted; grieves alone or silently. Deep sighing is a main symptom.

Modalities

Worse: touch; coffee, candy, tobacco. Better: deep breathing; swallowing, and eating.

Food/drink

Desires: fruit, sour food. Aversions: fruit, meat, milk, tobacco smoke.

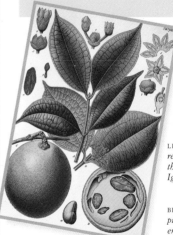

LEFT *The* Ignatia amara *remedy is prepared from the seeds of the St. Ignatius' bean plant.*

BELOW *The* Ign. *mental picture is one of deep emotional upset, often caused by loss.*

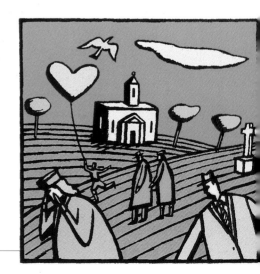

COMPLAINTS

❖ Headache
Head pains as if a nail is being driven into the brain, but it is relieved by lying on the painful side. Tension or migraine headaches after emotional experiences.

❖ Ear noise
Roaring sound in the ears, better when music is played.

❖ Cough
Dry, spasmodic, occurring in rapid bouts. Coughing makes the cough worse. Coughs when standing still, rather than when walking.

❖ Sore throat
Feeling that there is a lump in the throat that cannot be swallowed, relieved by eating something solid. Any feeling of lump in the throat. Choking sensation in throat.

❖ Digestive disorders
Appetite for different things, but no inclination to eat them when they are offered. Hunger with nausea. Empty, sinking feeling in the stomach that does not go away after eating. Nausea or vomiting that improves after eating indigestible things.

❖ Bowel disorders, hemorrhoids
Stool is painful and difficult, though soft; painful constriction in anus after the stool is passed. Hemorrhoids feel better for sitting.

❖ Urine retention
Urge, but inability, to pass urine.

❖ Insomnia
Light sleeper; every sound wakes. Recurring horrid dreams. Insomnia from grief, worry. Violent yawning, with emotional picture.

❖ Fever
Thirsty when chilled, but not thirsty when hot. Acute illnesses, such as tonsillitis, come on directly after a deep emotional shock.

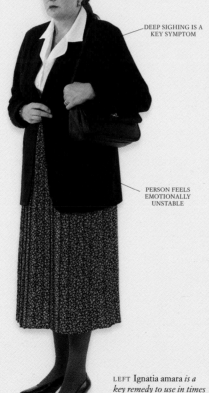

DEEP SIGHING IS A KEY SYMPTOM

PERSON FEELS EMOTIONALLY UNSTABLE

LEFT Ignatia amara *is a key remedy to use in times of bereavement or grief.*

NAT-M.

Like *Ign.*, *Nat-m.* is an important remedy after an experience of emotional upset, especially grief from loss. The person is more likely to hold in emotions, preferring to be alone to cry. Comfort from others results in even more distress or anger, unless comforted by the "right" person. For someone who appears calm on the surface, but responds passionately or overreacts to an insignificant event. Reactions indicating *Ign.* are contradictory or inappropriate; those of *Nat-m.* result from controlling emotions.

STAPH.

Complaints after a deep disappointment, with feelings of being insulted, humiliated, or injured. The feelings may not be openly expressed, but suppressed or rationalized.

83

Ipecacuanha
[IP.]

Ipecacuanha is derived from the Cephaelis ipecacuanha, a perennial plant native to Brazil. To make the remedy, the roots are dried, powdered, and either triturated or mixed with alcohol to make a tincture. It is used primarily for nausea and abdominal pains.

CONFIRMATION

Plant: CEPHAELIS IPECACUANHA *ipecac root*

WORSE
food

WORSE
warmth

THIRST
absent

BETTER
open air

- Nausea with any pain or problem
- Increased saliva
- No thirst
- Spasmodic cough

General indications
This remedy is primarily useful when nauseous symptoms predominate. Any combination of gastric and respiratory symptoms together. Nausea accompanies other complaints, such as profuse bleeding. Complaints may start after the person becomes angry or overeats. Rapid onset. Face pale or blue from inability to breathe.

Mental and emotional state
Sulky, cross; despises everything, and thinks others should too. Children are hard to please, crying and screaming for what they want; extremely impatient.

RIGHT *Ip. is an ideal remedy for nausea, especially in the early months of pregnancy.*

Modalities
Worse: smell of food; fatty meat, rich food, ice cream, fruit, coffee; warmth, humidity; cold and heat; cold, dry weather.
Better: open air; cold drinks (improve cough).

Food/drink
Desires: delicacies, candies.
Aversions: food (lack of appetite); drinks.
Thirst: none.

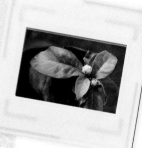

ABOVE *The* Ipecacuanha *plant grows in the tropical rainforests of Central and South America.*

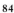

COMPLAINTS

❖ Headache
With a bruised feeling; with nausea. Gastric headache. Migraine with nausea and vomiting.

❖ Common cold
Nose is blocked at night, then hoarse cough comes on with retching and vomiting.

❖ Cough
Frequently indicated in cough with nausea in children. The child stiffens, and becomes red or blue in the face, nauseous, and vomits. Constant and violent cough; gasping for breath. Cough causes vomiting, without nausea. Dry, spasmodic cough ends in choking and gagging. Loose, coarse rattling in the chest, but no phlegm is brought up. Nosebleed from cough, with nausea. Difficulty in breathing. Feeling of constriction in the chest, which is worse for movement.

❖ Abdominal pain, nausea
Nausea with profuse salivation. Constant, distressing nausea; inclination to vomit, but nausea is not relieved by vomiting. Need to bring up wind; empty belching. Stomach pains after extreme anger. Griping, cutting, colicky pain around the navel, made worse from movement.

❖ Diarrhea
Frequent diarrhea of green, slimy stool, after sour or unripe fruit. Appears frothy, fermented.

❖ Fever
Chill alternating with heat. No thirst while hot. Constant nausea.

CHILDREN
Refer to coughs (*See above*).

WOMEN

❖ Vomiting and Nausea
In pregnancy. Bleeding from uterus with nausea; nausea during labor.

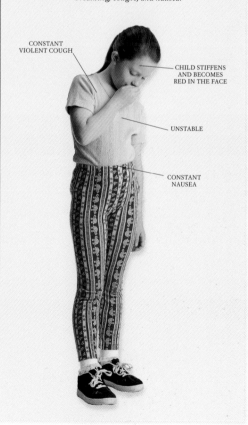

BELOW *The symptom picture for* Ip. *includes difficulty in breathing, coughs, and nausea.*

CONSTANT VIOLENT COUGH

CHILD STIFFENS AND BECOMES RED IN THE FACE

UNSTABLE

CONSTANT NAUSEA

COMPARISON OF REMEDIES

NAUSEA IN PREGNANCY

CIMIC.
Nausea with depressed emotions, feeling of gloom and pessimism; worse for cold and damp weather, better for keeping warm.

KALI BIC.
Vomiting of bright yellow water during pregnancy. Mucous membranes generally affected; chilly person.

PULS.
Vomiting of mucus during pregnancy. Warm person, desiring open windows, doors, or being in the open air. Emotional, affectionate, clingy, craves sympathy.

SEP.
Nausea – desires to be alone, sense of detachment, does not like consolation. Chilly, desires warmth.

Kali bichromium

[KALI BIC.]

Kali bichromium *is prepared from potassium bichromate. Granules are triturated, or dissolved in purified water. It is mainly used homeopathically to treat discharges from the mucous membranes from the nose, throat, vagina, urethra, and stomach. It is a good remedy for sinusitis.*

General indications

This remedy primarily affects the mucous membranes of nose, throat, lungs, stomach, and intestines. Onset is slow and affects deeply. Person becomes weak and weary. Discharges of mucus are thick, sticky, stringy or lumpy, ropey, yellow. There may be a yellowish coating on the tongue, or yellow eyewhites, vomit, or phlegm. Person usually prone to catarrh, especially in sinuses. Pains, felt in small spots, may come and go quickly, or move quickly from place to place. Rheumatic joint pains. Chilly people who catch cold easily.

Mental and emotional state

Avoids mental or physical labor.

Modalities

Worse: cold damp weather; spring; and fall, 2–3 a.m.
Better: heat, motion.

Food/drink

Desires: beer, acid drinks.
Aversions: meat (indigestible).

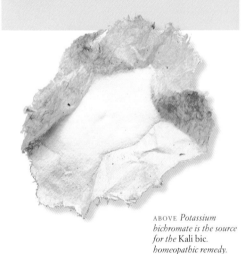

ABOVE *Potassium bichromate is the source for the* Kali bic. *homeopathic remedy.*

BELOW Kali bic. *is given for complaints that affect the mucous membranes.*

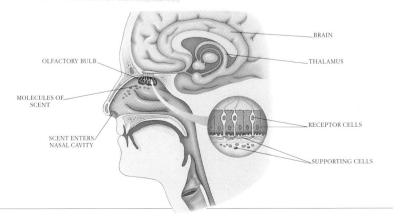

BRAIN

THALAMUS

OLFACTORY BULB

MOLECULES OF SCENT

RECEPTOR CELLS

SCENT ENTERS NASAL CAVITY

SUPPORTING CELLS

COMPLAINTS

❖ **Headache**
Migraine; head pain in small spots, with blindness or dim vision. Occurs at the same time every day.

❖ **Earache**
With thick, yellow, smelly discharge. Especially the left side.

❖ **Common cold**
Sinusitis. Nose feels stuffed with a sensation of pressure and fullness at upper part of nose; dry. Sinus pain, over and along the eyebrows, feels better for pressing the top part of the nose. Discharge is thick, green or yellow, smelly, and causes soreness of the skin around the nose. The thick mucus forms crusts that are difficult to remove, leaving the skin raw.

❖ **Sore throat**
Dry and rough; the throat looks red, shiny, and puffy. Tonsils inflamed, with deep ulcers. Brings up much tough, thick, sticky mucus from throat. Voice is rough and hoarse.

❖ **Cough**
Cough, from tickling in larynx, is worse after eating. Coughs up the characteristic phlegm – thick, yellow, sticky, stringy, profuse. Metallic, hacking cough in croup. There may be pain from the front of the chest to the back, between the shoulderblades.

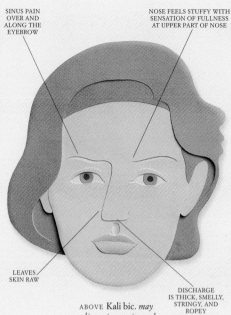

SINUS PAIN OVER AND ALONG THE EYEBROW

NOSE FEELS STUFFY WITH SENSATION OF FULLNESS AT UPPER PART OF NOSE

LEAVES SKIN RAW

DISCHARGE IS THICK, SMELLY, STRINGY, AND ROPEY

ABOVE Kali bic. *may relieve sinus pain, and help blocked noses.*

❖ **Digestive disorders**
Dry mouth. Vomiting of bright yellow water or mucus. Complaints are better for eating. Complaints from drinking too much beer, vomiting after drinking beer.

❖ **Diarrhea**
Brown, frothy. Diarrhea from drinking beer. Painful pressure in rectum.

❖ **Aches and pains**
Pains move from place to place. Worse for changes of weather or cold air. Back pain at base of spine.

WOMEN

❖ **Vomiting**
During pregnancy.

❖ **Thrush**
Yellow, ropey, sticky discharge from vagina.

MEN

❖ **Urinary disorders**
Constriction at root of penis. Stinging, profuse discharge, jellylike discharge blocks the urethra. Pain in prostate forces him to stand still; worse for walking. Prostatitis.

COMPARISON OF REMEDIES

FOR MUCOUS DISCHARGE

MERC.
Discharges from mucous membranes are green, or green/yellow, causing soreness and rawness of the skin; more foul smelling than *Kali bic.* Glands are usually affected, swollen. Profuse sweat accompanies many complaints. Sensitive to both extremes of hot and cold; only better in a moderate temperature.

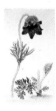

PULS.
Mucous membrane discharges are thick, yellow, and bland; from eyes, nose, ears, urethra, etc. Warm person who prefers cool, open air. Symptoms change frequently – shifting sides of the body, or location. Emotional, craves sympathy, often weepy and clingy. Not usually thirsty.

87

Lachesis

[LACH.]

Lachesis *is prepared from the fresh venom of the bushmaster snake, a native of the South American continent. The venom is triturated to make the remedy. It is used homeopathically to treat circulatory problems, menopausal problems, and left-sided symptoms.*

General indications
Lachesis primarily affects the mind, blood circulation, throat, and ovaries. Onset is intense and rapid. Hemorrhages; flushes of heat; oozing of diarrhea. Complaints may come on during, or just after, sleep. Sensation that there is a lump in various parts of the body. Feelings of constriction. Intense emotions. Effects of injuries and puncture wounds. Blue skin around bites, or inflamed spots. Menopausal symptoms. Left-sided.

Mental and emotional state
Very talkative and jumps from one subject to another. Sharp-tongued. Overactive mind. Free expression through language, which is used as a weapon – jesting, tactless, satirical. Intense, extreme emotions. Person may be jealous, suspicious, paranoid; exuberant, excitable, exhilarated. Complaints from grief or disappointed love. Depressed and anxious in the morning after waking. Complaints come on during or just after sleep; for this reason person may dread going to sleep.

Modalities
Worse: sleep; heat, summer, sun; empty swallowing; slight touch or pressure; alcohol. Better: open air; free discharges; hard pressure; cold drinks.

Food/drink
Desires: alcoholic drinks, oysters, coffee. Aversions: warm food, bread, tobacco.

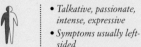

CONFIRMATION

Snake: CROTALUS MUTUS *surukuku, deadly bushmaster*

WORSE
heat

WORSE
on left side

BETTER
cold drinks

BETTER
open air

- *Talkative, passionate, intense, expressive*
- *Symptoms usually left-sided*
- *Warm*
- *Purple discoloration*
- *Complaints during or after sleep*

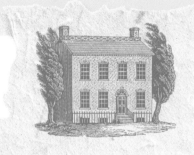

BELOW *The deadly poisonous bushmaster snake is the source for* Lachesis.

ABOVE *The* Lachesis *patient feels better for fresh air and being out in the open.*

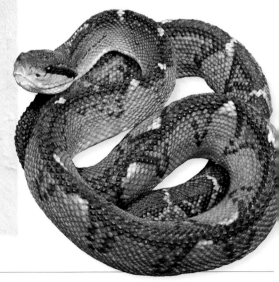

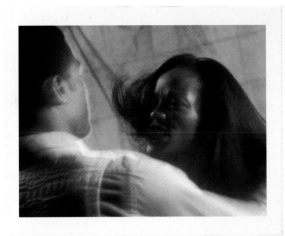

BELL.
Excited, delirious; acute senses; sudden onset of inflammations with dryness, redness, and heat.

PULS.
Mild, gentle disposition, seeks cool air.

LEFT *A* Lachesis *trait is aggression, when the person openly expresses jealousy or suspicion.*

COMPLAINTS

❖ **Headache**
Head feels heavy, bursting, as if all the blood has gone to the head. Hammering, pulsating headache. Migraine, with pain extending to neck and shoulders. Head aches from exposure to the sun, or drinking too much alcohol.

❖ **Nosebleed**
From blowing the nose, with dark blood.

❖ **Mouth affections**
Gums are bluish, swollen, bleed easily. Bad breath. Thick saliva.

❖ **Sore throat**
Purplish dark color. Feeling that there is a lump in the throat that comes up, but goes down again. Sensation of suffocation, as if there were something swollen in the throat. Throat pain extends to the ears. Swallowing is very painful, but throat feels better when swallowing solids, and worse when swallowing liquids or nothing at all. Worse for hot drinks. Externally, throat is very sensitive to touch; person cannot bear anything around the neck. Left side is especially affected.

❖ **Cough**
Person must take deep breaths. Touching the neck causes a tickling, choking cough. Coughs during sleep without waking; worse during sleep. Feeling of suffocation on lying down to go to sleep.

❖ **Fever**
Heat at the top of the head; flushes of heat on falling asleep. Chill stage is worse for drinking.

❖ **Skin injuries, sores**
Injuries bleed freely, oozing dark red blood. Sores are purple/bluish around the edges as are bedsores, boils, infected ulcers.

❖ **Joint pain**
Purple discoloration around the joints, which are swollen and hot.

WOMEN

❖ **Symptoms of menopause**
Palpitations and flushes of heat, with headache (*see headache*); fainting. Nosebleed during menopause.

❖ **Hair loss**
During pregnancy.

SPECIAL
APPLICATIONS
Sunstroke: Face is dark red or bluish after extreme heat; rushes of blood to the head; worse after sleep.

Ledum

[LED.]

This remedy is prepared from the wild rosemary shrub, which is found in Europe and Canada. The whole fresh plant is pounded, steeped in alcohol, then strained and filtered to make the tincture. It is used as a first aid remedy for puncture wounds and joint pain.

General indications
Ledum **affects skin, small joints such as ankles and wrists, and tendons. Swelling, numbness, pain, and cold. Person gets cold and chilly, but the parts affected are better when treated with cold applications and the person feels better generally from a cool environment.** *Ledum* **can prevent tetanus if taken immediately after a deep puncture wound.**

Mental and emotional state
No marked symptoms.

Modalities
Worse: warmth; movement of affected part; night. Better: cold; rest, keeping the part still.

Food/drink
Desires: alcoholic drinks, which makes symptoms worse.

BELOW *The night tends to make symptoms worse for the Ledum patient.*

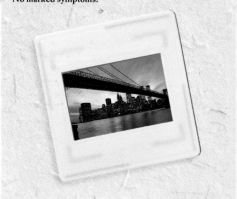

CONFIRMATION

Plant: LEDUM PALUSTRE *wild rosemary, marsh tea*

WORSE
warmth

WORSE
movement

WORSE
at night

BETTER
cold

- *Injuries to skin, joints, with swelling*
- *Skin feels cold to the touch*
- *Better for cold applications or treatments*
- *Worse for warmth of bed, application of heat externally*

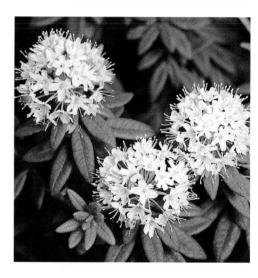

ABOVE *Wild rosemary has antiseptic properties that helps prevent tetanus.*

COMPLAINTS

❖ **Eye affections**
Bloodshot, bruised; black eye from injury.

❖ **Joint pain**
Stiffness. Sprained ankles. Soles painful, preventing walking. Person cannot lift feet from the ground; wants to soak the feet in cold water. Joints rheumatic: puffy, purple, cold. Acute rheumatic pain when the joint is swollen and hot but not red. Knees trembly, weak, with a shooting pain that is made worse by walking. The big toe joint is affected. The parts are cold to the touch but the person feels they are hot.

❖ **Wounds, bites**
Puncture wounds that feel cold or bleed little. Injury such as stepping on a nail. Stings. Black-and-blue swelling, red spots, rash. Animal bites. Affected area very sensitive to the touch, becomes septic. Always feels better from cold applications and worse from heat.

COMPARISON OF REMEDIES

APIS
Insect bites and stings when the skin becomes red, hot, shiny, and swollen. Also for joints that become swollen, hot, and red. In both cases the pains are stinging and burning, worse for any form of warmth and better for cold bathing or applications. Hives with red raised patches and intense itching, with the same modalities.

ARN.
The first remedy to consider for trauma or any injury, with mental and/or physical shock. The person does not want to be touched or even approached for fear of being touched, and may deny anything is wrong. Either the whole body or a part feels sore and bruised. Not to be used topically on open wounds.

CAL.
Used topically as an antiseptic, and to accelerate new growth of skin. For cuts, grazes, lacerations, and in the later stages of burns, after the blisters have burst. Soothes and promotes healing of injuries to skin.

HYP.
The first remedy to consider in cases of damage to nerves and nerve-rich tissues, and penetrating wounds such as those caused by needles. With sharp, shooting pains, tingling and/or numbness.

LACH.
For animal bites or other skin injuries where there is bluish/purplish discoloration of the skin or oozing of dark red blood. Joint injuries with swelling, blue/purple mottled appearance. Warm person, where the skin feels warm to touch, and are worse from heat, touch, and slight pressure, better from cold and hard pressure.

RHUS T.
Sprains and strains of joints that are better from heat and worse from cold and damp. The part affected is stiff and painful on first moving, but eases up and feels better after continued motion. A feeling of restlessness, inability to remain still is an important indication for *Rhus-t.*

RUTA
For injuries to cartilage, ligaments, bones, not as much muscle or tendon. The damage is deeper into the joint. Sore, bruised pain better for warmth and movement, worse for cold and damp.

LEFT Ledum
*is a useful first
aid remedy for
puncture wounds.*

Lycopodium

[LYC.]

Club moss is the source plant for Lycopodium. *It grows in mountains and forests of the Northern Hemisphere. To prepare the homeopathic remedy, the crushed spores are steeped in alcohol, the mixture is then strained and filtered. It is used to treat digestive disorders.*

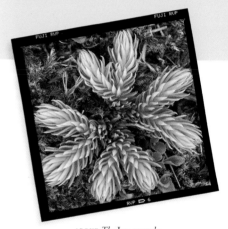

CONFIRMATION

Plant: LYCOPODIUM CLAVATUM *club moss*

WORSE
warmth

WORSE
4–8 p.m.

BETTER
warm drinks

BETTER
movement

- *Desires candy, hot drinks*
- *Worse 4–8 p.m.*
- *Symptoms mental more than physical*
- *Flatulence, fullness after eating*
- *Pains predominantly right-sided, but can move from right to left*

ABOVE *The* Lyc. *remedy is made from the flowering spikes of the club moss.*

General indications
Lycopodium **primarily affects the digestive system, the liver, and the urinary system. Person feels full of gas, inflated. Complaints develop gradually. Symptoms are predominantly right-sided, but may move from right to left, especially in throat complaints. Tends to be cold and dry. Desires candy.**

Mental and emotional state
Sensitive, fearful, afraid to be alone; likes someone nearby. Strong and domineering outwardly, and/or timid, lacking in self-confidence. Anticipates an ordeal, becomes nervous before a test or public appearance. Does not like doing anything new.

Modalities
Worse: warmth; pressure of clothes; milk, vegetables, cabbage, beans, bread, pastry, cold food; 4–8 p.m. Better: warm drinks; moving around; belching.

Food/drink
Desires: candy, hot food, olives, alcohol. Aversions: beans, peas, cabbage (causing flatulence).

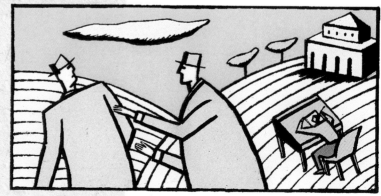

RIGHT *The* Lyc. *patient does not want to be alone and has a fear of exams.*

COMPLAINTS

❖ Emotional problems
Anxiety before important events, e.g. exams, public appearances, caused by fear of inadequate performance (though this is usually proved to be unfounded). Sleepless from worry about the outcome of an event, such as an examination.

❖ Headache
Headache caused by, or worse for, not eating properly, or mental strain. Catarrhal headache over eyes with severe colds. Pain moves from the right side to the left.

❖ Common cold
Headache in forehead; sinuses and nose blocked with yellow catarrh, making it necessary to breathe through the mouth. Nose blocked but dry, worse on the right side. Small amount of burning discharge, forming crusts and elastic plugs.

❖ Sore throat
Extremely painful; better for drinking warm drinks, and swallowing. Swollen, ulcerated tonsils. Starts on right side of throat an moves to the left.

❖ Ear complaints
Humming, roaring noises; blockage causing deafness. Discharge may be sticky, thick, yellow, offensive (glue ear).

❖ Cough
Dry, tickling, teasing cough. Short, rattling breathing made worse by lying on the back, yawning, and breathing deeply. Cough produces salty, greenish-yellow, lumpy or foul phlegm. Craves air.

❖ Digestive disorders
Hunger satisfied after a few mouthfuls. Eating a little creates a feeling of fullness. Heartburn or indigestion with bitter burping, rises to the throat. Anxiety felt in stomach. Noisy flatulence. Fullness, distension, bloating. Abdomen is sensitive to the least pressure, causing the person to loosen clothing.

❖ Constipation
Feels as if stool remains in rectum; there is no desire to pass stool, though the rectum is full. Particularly constipated when away from home.

❖ Cystitis
Urine retention; urine slow in coming – must strain. Copious urination at night. Pressing feeling in bladder and abdomen. Constant bearing down feeling. Urine milky, bloody, or with red sediment.

CHILDREN

❖ Snuffles
In babies. Difficulty breathing/nursing; must breathe through mouth.

❖ Colic
Worse in the evening, with distension; worse for heat, tightly fitting diapers or clothes.

❖ Urinary affections
Child cries before passing urine.

BELOW Lyc. *symptoms include colic in babies, which may be aggravated by tight-fitting diapers.*

ARG-N.
Much more impulsive and hurried. Nervous diarrhea.

COLOC.
Better for bending double, drawing up limbs, hard pressure on stomach.

SIL.
Yielding but extremely sensitive. Perspires easily, especially on the head and feet. Chilly and thirsty.

Magnesium phosphoricum

[MAG-P.]

Magnesium phosphoricum *is made by mixing magnesium sulfate and sodium phosphate in water. The crystals formed are then triturated. It is used homeopathically to relieve spasms and cramps, including menstrual pain.*

CONFIRMATION

Mineral: MAGNESIUM PHOSPHATE

SENSITIVE
to pain

THIRST
cold drinks

BETTER
warmth

WORSE
on right side

- *Always talking of pains*
- *Excruciating neuralgia, cramping pains*
- *Worse for cold, better for heat, hard pressure*

General indications
Pain from irritation of nerves (neuralgia), and spasms. Pains are violent, excruciating, maddening, cutting, stinging, cramping, griping; better for hard pressure and heat. Chilly; worse for cold, better for heat. Tiredness, exhaustion. Cramps from overexertion.

Mental and emotional state
Always talking and lamenting about the pain.

Modalities
Worse: right side; touch; cold of any kind, such as wind, bath, night, milk.
Better: warmth, hot bathing; pressure.

Food/drink
Desires: very cold drinks.
No marked aversions.

BELOW *Mag-p. is made from magnesium phosphate, a tissue salt present in parts of the human body.*

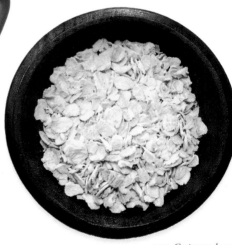

LEFT *Grain cereals are a rich source of magnesium phosphate.*

LEFT *The symptom picture for Mag-p. includes violent spasms and cramps, with a griping pain.*

COMPLAINTS

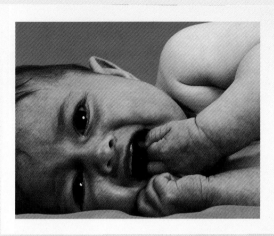

ABOVE *Use* Mag-p. *as a remedy for teething pain to help soothe babies' sore, inflamed gums.*

❖ **Headache**
Neuralgic headache, throbbing; better for wrapping up tightly (pressure), warm compresses, warm room.

❖ **Face pains**
Neuralgia on the right side; worse from any cold.

❖ **Eye complaints**
Shooting, stinging, shifting spasmodic pain; sparks before eyes.

❖ **Toothache**
Better for heat, hot fluids in the mouth. Teething in children.

❖ **Digestive disorders**
Spasms, cramps in stomach. Pain is griping, pinching, and not relieved by belching. Cramp feels as if there is a tight band around the body. Colic caused by flatulence, causes the person to bend double, which relieves the pain. Better for warmth, rubbing, pressure. Bloated fullness in abdomen; person must loosen the clothes and walk around.

❖ **Muscle cramps**
Cramps, caused by overuse of hands, fingers, etc., with characteristic modalities as above.

CHILDREN

❖ **Colic**
Causes the legs to be drawn up.

❖ **Teething**
Painful teething, better for warmth externally.

WOMEN

❖ **Menstrual pain**
Relieved by external heat and pressure applied to the abdomen.

CAUTION

Chronic menstrual problems should be treated constitutionally by a homeopath.

CHAM.
Intolerable pains of physical complaints with an angry, ugly mood, where the person is temperamental and oversensitive. Children will want to be carried and demand many things, but then push them away when offered. Adults in this state become argumentative, snappy, or abusive to those around. Screaming, shrieking with pain.

COLOC.
Abdominal cramps with sudden, forceful, cutting, or gnawing pains. Colic, indigestion caused by an experience of overexcitement or anger; or from eating unripe fruit or drinking unclean water. The pains are relieved by bending over double, or pressing hard on the abdomen. Passing wind brings temporary relief.

NUX V.
Complaints after overeating and/or drinking too much alcohol. The stomach feels too full, with indigestion, nausea; headache with dull pain and dizziness. Abdomen is bloated and worse for any pressure, must loosen clothing around the waist. The person wants to vomit, would be relieved by vomiting, but cannot. Irritable, oversensitive, and overstimulated like *Cham.*, but chillier and less thirsty. This combination of symptoms resembles the picture of a typical hangover.

Mercurius

[MERC.]

The Mercurius *remedy is made by mixing mercury oxide with nitric acid. It is used to treat symptoms that are sensitive to both heat and cold and when the state of illness is similar to a toxic state.*

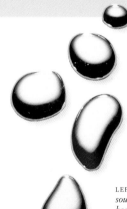
General indications

Mercurius **mainly affects glands (lymph, salivary, and throat), tonsils, and mucous membranes. Pus and/or ulcerations, swelling, increased secretions. Profuse discharges: drenching sweat with many complaints; copious saliva. Foul, offensive breath. Secretions may be thin, acrid, burning, and foul, or thick, green-yellow, and cause soreness and rawness of the skin. Easily chilled and overheated; very sensitive to changes in temperature.**

Mental and emotional state

Very closed; difficult to make contact. Discontented. Changeable, but feels worse for the change.

Modalities

**Worse: night, night air; damp, cold, or heat (warm bed, fire, room); sweating (does not bring relief); worse lying on right side.
Better: moderate temperatures; lying on abdomen; rest; morning.**

Food/drink

**Desires: bread and butter, cold drinks.
Aversions: salty, rich foods, candy.
Thirst: intense, for large amounts of water, despite copious saliva.**

BELOW *The* Merc. *symptom picture may include an aversion to salty foods.*

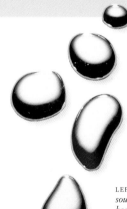

LEFT *Mercury is the source for the* Mercurius *homeopathic remedy.*

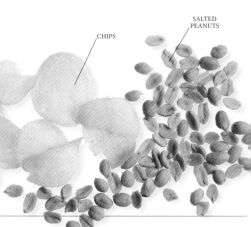

ANCHOVIES

CHIPS

SALTED PEANUTS

COMPLAINTS

❖ **Headache**
Tension in scalp, as if bandaged; feeling as if head is in a vise.

❖ **Eye affections**
Cannot stand light. Eyes are watery with burning discharge; inflammation with mucus or pus. Worse for cold, heat of bed.

❖ **Earache**
External inflammation, and internal (otitis media). Great pain, cramping, stitching. Bloody, foul, smelly discharge from ear. Pains extend to ear from teeth and throat.

❖ **Common cold**
Violent sneezing, and discharge of green, corrosive mucus, smelling of old cheese.

❖ **Mouth disorders, toothache**
Salivary glands are painful and swollen; saliva profuse. Odd tastes or sensations in the mouth such as salty, sweet, metallic, slimy. Swollen, flabby tongue; bleeding gums; offensive breath. Teeth feel as if they are loose, painful. Violent toothache, with chilliness.

❖ **Sore throat**
Dry; tonsils are inflamed and ulcerated, with shooting pains, and exude pus. Swallowing painful; tonsils deep red, swollen; worse for hot or cold drinks.

❖ **Diarrhea**
With green mucus; feels as if never completely done. Changeable stool. Diarrhea with sensitivity to changes in temperature. Travelers' diarrhea. Painful straining to pass stool.

❖ **Fevers**
Fever with stomach upsets; very sweaty during sleep. Strong odors. Chills and heat alternate. Perspiration does not relieve.

CHILDREN

❖ **Chicken pox**
Vesicles exude pus.

❖ **Mumps**
Worse on right side. Offensive salivation; foul tongue; sweat.

ARS.
Colds with thin, watery, fluent, burning discharge from the nose. Generally very chilly and thirsty, with burning pains better for heat. Restless, frequently changing positions; may be overly fussy, fault finding, or concerned with detail. Also digestive problems as from food poisoning.

HEP.
Swollen tonsils and glands of the neck with pains as if a splinter is stuck in the throat. Extreme sensitivity to pain as well as to the least external influence such as touch, noise, flow of air. Better for keeping warm, moist warmth, and covering. Discharges will be offensive, as in *Merc.*, but the pain and sensitivity of *Hep.* are more acute.

PHYT.
Glands inflamed. Sharp pains appear and disappear suddenly. Ulcerated tonsils; throat feels better for cold drinks. Feeling of a lump in the throat. Think of this remedy for affections of the glands – breasts, tonsils, etc. – with aching, hardness, and swelling, without clearly marked mental/ emotional symptoms.

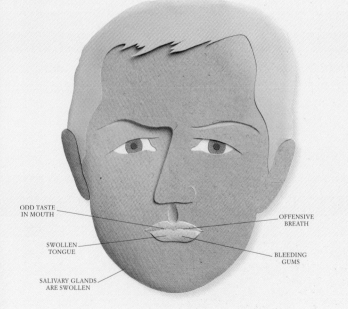

ODD TASTE
IN MOUTH

OFFENSIVE
BREATH

SWOLLEN
TONGUE

BLEEDING
GUMS

SALIVARY GLANDS
ARE SWOLLEN

LEFT Merc. *is a useful remedy for mouth and throat complaints.*

Natrum muriaticum

[NAT-M.]

This remedy is prepared from rock salt,
or common table salt. Pure salt crystals are
triturated with lactose sugar to prepare the
homeopathic remedy. It is used to treat
emotional upsets, particularly suppressed grief.

CONFIRMATION

Mineral: SODIUM CHLORIDE *common table salt*

WORSE
9–11 a. m.

WORSE
sun

WORSE
movement (exercise)

THIRST
all drinks

- Dryness; watery discharges; thirst.
- Worse in the morning, when the sun comes up, and for exposure to sun.
- Complaints after grief.
- Desires salt, or salty foods.

General indications

Many of the proving physical symptoms are similar to those in people who take too much salt in their diet. Easily fatigued, with physical and mental weakness. Because the balance of water in the system is disturbed, symptoms may alternate: a person may suffer from dryness of lips, skin, stool, or mucous membranes, with great thirst; or profuse watery discharges. *Natrum muriaticum* is an important remedy for symptoms that result from an emotional upset, especially grief.

Mental and emotional state

Sad, depressed, weepy, but consolation causes more distress, even anger, unless comforted by the right person. The person may appear calm, preferring to cry alone. Broods about unpleasant events. Insignificant events may trigger a passionate response.

Modalities

Worse: in the morning, 9–11 a.m.; from exposure to the sun; before menses; after eating; physical exertion. Better: after sweating; rest.

Food/drink

Desires: bitter or salty food. Aversions: bread, and anything slimy, such as oysters or fat. Thirst: unquenchable.

BELOW *Nat-m. people can only be comforted by the right person.*

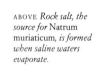

ABOVE *Rock salt, the source for* Natrum muriaticum, *is formed when saline waters evaporate.*

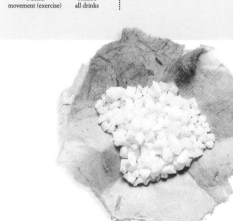

COMPLAINTS

❖ Emotional problems
Feelings of sadness or grief, but cannot cry. Acute circumstances only.

❖ Headache
Blinding headache, as if a thousand hammers were knocking on the brain. Starts in the morning, after waking. Eyes sore and watery. Worse for the heat of the sun, coughing, and for any kind of mental activity such as reading or thinking. Comes on after experience of grief, during or after the menstrual period, with nausea and vomiting. Better for firm pressure on the head, and for sleep.

❖ Cold sores
Around the mouth, on lower lip, on corners of the mouth, which appear after exposure to the sun, or after grief that was not expressed. Lips dry, with a crack in the middle of lower lip.

❖ Common cold
Cold starts with forceful sneezing. Nasal discharge of thin, watery catarrh, like the white of an egg, then nose becomes completely dry and blocked. Dryness alternates with fluent catarrh. Loss of taste and smell. With cold sores and/or headache (see above). Symptoms are worse in the fresh air. With characteristic mental and general symptoms.

❖ Indigestion, heartburn
Indigestion, when emotional state affects the stomach. Heartburn and acidic belching that is difficult, incomplete, and does not make the person feel better. There is a bitter or salty taste in the mouth. The person is hungry, but does not enjoy food, or prefers not to eat, feeling better on an empty stomach. Abdomen distended, with cutting pains (gas pains).

❖ Constipation
Hard, dry, crumbly stool that is difficult to pass. Feels that there is more stool in rectum.

❖ Urine retention
Action of bladder is slow. Must wait for urine to start. A peculiar symptom is that the person is unable to urinate in a public toilet.

❖ Fever
Intermittent fever. (This remedy is used as prophylaxis for malaria.) With headache, hot face, thirst. Drinks often and a lot. Nausea and vomiting; blurred vision; feeling faint. Fever without chill. Worse 10–11 a.m. Or: chill with thirst, severe headache, nausea and vomiting, extreme cold internally. Symptoms occur at the same time every day.

SPECIAL APPLICATIONS
Sunstroke: heat in head, red face, nausea and vomiting, head feels as if it would burst; blinding of eyes, sees zigzags. After malaria or misuse of quinine, when symptoms agree.

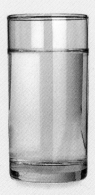

LEFT *The symptom picture for* Nat-m. *includes an unquenchable thirst.*

COMPARISON OF REMEDIES

BELL.
Sudden onset, high temperature, inflammations, affections of the brain.

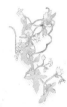

BRY.
Slow onset of inflammations. All complaints are much worse for any movements.

IGN.
Emotional outbursts, sighing; worse for open air. Emotionally contradictary and alternating states; aversion to fruit and tobacco smoke

Nux vomica

[NUX V.]

Nux vomica *is prepared from the seeds of the* Strychnos nux vomica *plant, which is native to Australia and the East Indies. The dried seeds are steeped in alcohol, then strained and filtered to make the tincture. It is used to treat digestive disorders, as well as colds and fevers.*

General indications
Digestive disturbances. Exaggerated sensitivity and irritability; extreme sensitivity to pain, or overstimulation. Fiery temperament, easily offended, quarrelsome, becomes aggressive, uncontrollably angry. There is a desire for stimulants, but these tend to make the person feel even worse.

Mental and emotional state
Very irritable, angry, and impatient. Hypochondriacal; talks about the illness. Aversion to noise, odors, light. Inability to stand the pain.

Modalities
Worse: early morning (4 a.m.); cold; high living, overindulgence in rich foods/alcohol; sedentary habits; mental exertion. Slight causes: touch, pressure of clothes. Better: free discharges; naps; hot drinks; milk; moist air; warm room, covering.

Food/drink
Desires: stimulants – alcohol, coffee, tobacco; food; fats. Aversions: ale, beer, coffee, food, meat, tobacco, water.

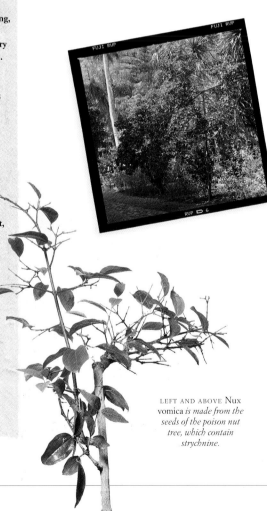

LEFT AND ABOVE Nux vomica *is made from the seeds of the poison nut tree, which contain strychnine.*

COMPLAINTS

❖ Headache
Intoxicated feeling; headache with squeezing, dull pain in top of head or over the eyes. Vertigo; brain feels as if it is turning a circle. Better for warm room, sitting quietly, lying down. Headache in the sunshine.

❖ Common cold
Profuse discharge during the day; stuffed up at night and out of doors. Stuffed up feeling; violent sneezing.

❖ Sore throat
Rough, scraped feeling. Tickling after waking in the morning. Sensation of roughness, tightness, tension. Pharynx constricted, uvula swollen, stitches into ear. Pain worse for empty swallowing.

❖ Cough
Cough causes bursting headache. Shallow breathing. Cough after mental effort; better for warm drinks, worse for physical exertion.

❖ Fever
Extreme chilliness; worse for slightest movement. Chilliness on being uncovered, but does not want to be covered. Chill and thirst; and headache without thirst.

BELOW *Overindulgence in unhealthy foods is common in the* Nux vomica *patient, although this will aggravate their symptoms.*

NUX V. TYPES LIKE FATTY FOODS

❖ Digestive disorders
Nausea; sour vomiting ailments from overeating and drinking. Stomach feels overloaded just after eating. Colic or indigestion causes nausea. Wants to vomit, but cannot. Flatulent distension just after eating. Hungry, yet averse to food. Weight and pain in stomach, very sensitive to pressure. Quickly better for rest, sitting, or lying. Pains are better for heat. Symptoms correspond to a typical hangover.

❖ Constipation/ diarrhea
Pains in rectum after a meal. Frequent, ineffectual desire to stool; passes small amounts each time and feels as if some remains. Diarrhea dark; in morning, or immediately after a meal.

COMPARISON OF REMEDIES

GENERAL

ARS.
Burning pains better for warmth. Unquenchable thirst. Desires company out of fear.

CHAM.
Irritable, oversensitive and angry mood, similar to *Nux v.,* but more emphasis on the intolerable pains that accompany complaints such as teething, colic, earache.

LYC.
Worse 4–8 p.m. Full of gas, flatulence, better for passing wind. Lack of self-confidence.

SUL.
Indigestion, colic, distended abdomen, with grumbling in the lower intestines. Generally warm, and worse for becoming heated. Better for open air, motion. Redness of eyelids, lips, anus. Diarrhea with teething.

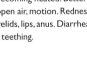

Phosphorus

[PHOS.]

Essential to life, the mineral Phosphorus *is found in all living matter. Now used primarily by homeopaths, it was once used in traditional medicine to treat malaria and epilepsy. It is triturated to prepare the homeopathic remedy.*

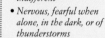

CONFIRMATION

Mineral: PHOSPHORUS

SENSATION
chilly

WORSE
touch, odors, light

WORSE
cold weather

BETTER
eating

- *Chilly*
- *Thirsty for cold drinks, which relieve pains*
- *Open, sensitive, impressionable, or indifferent*
- *Nervous, fearful when alone, in the dark, or of thunderstorms*

General indications
Phosphorus **affects all tissues and functions, especially nutrition, blood, and the mucous membranes of the respiratory and digestive tracts. The homeopathic picture has irritations and inflammations. Burning pains. Suffering from lack of food: must eat or will faint. Hemorrhages. Small wounds bleed profusely with bright red blood. Blood-streaked discharges. Persistent bleeding; blood does not coagulate. Usually chilly, but craves coolness and cold drinks.**

Mental and emotional state
Affectionate, sympathetic, sensitive to surroundings. Wants sympathy, company, touch, physical contact. Also the opposite: not caring, indifferent. Fearful and anxious. Very impressionable, full of imaginings. Fears being alone, especially during thunderstorms.

Modalities
Worse: emotions, talking, touch, odors, light. Warm food; mental fatigue; cold weather, thunderstorms; lying on the left side. Better: eating; sleep; cold food and water; cold water on the face.

Food/drink
Desires: cold drinks and food, ice cream, spicy and salty food. Aversions: fruit, warm food and drink, garlic, onions, coffee. Thirst: very thirsty for iced water.

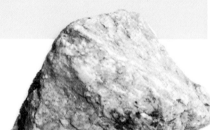

ABOVE *An adult's skeleton contains over 3lb (1.4kg) of* Phosphorus, *which is essential for the body's well-being.*

LEFT Phos. *is a useful remedy for treating malfunctions of cellular or tissue metabolism.*

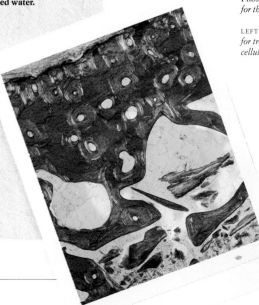

COMPLAINTS

❖ Headache
Headache from fasting. Dull pain, throbbing with sensation of heat. Better for cold air, washing face with cold water, cold compress to forehead.

❖ Common cold
Dull headache over one eye. Laryngitis with violent tickle in voice box; hoarse voice, tight chest, catarrh in lungs. Profuse, thin nasal discharge; when dry, crusts form and adhere to nostrils. One nostril discharges, the other is blocked; or dryness alternates with fluid, blood-streaked coryza. Mucous membranes of nose become swollen and feel stuffed. Nose blocked, better in open air. Profuse yellow-green discharge; blowing blood from nose.

❖ Sore throat
Tonsils swollen with a dry, burning sensation; worse for going from warm to cold air (room). Sneezing causes pain in throat. Loss of voice from nervous, emotional cause, or overstrain of voice. Acute laryngitis combined with dry, tickly cough.

❖ Cough
Dry, tickly irritation in larynx or upper chest. Hard, dry, tight cough that is exhausting, violent (forceful), and causes trembling. Feeling of weight on chest. Coughs up salty, yellow and/or bright red or rust colored, sour or sweet sputum. Using the voice or laughing worsens the cough. Cough causes burning in air passages.

❖ Fever
Flushed cheeks, especially left side. Hot and sweaty at night; very hungry. Profuse perspiration over whole body. No thirst.

❖ Digestive disorders
Inflammation of stomach; burning pains extend to throat and bowel. Nausea from warm drinks. Cold drinks, food, ice cream relieve pains. Cold water vomited when warm in stomach. Vomiting after surgery (from the effects of anesthetic).

❖ Diarrhea
Painless, profuse, exhausting, pouring out. Worse in the morning

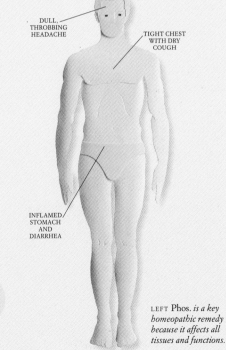

DULL, THROBBING HEADACHE

TIGHT CHEST WITH DRY COUGH

INFLAMED STOMACH AND DIARRHEA

LEFT *Phos. is a key homeopathic remedy because it affects all tissues and functions.*

COMPARISON OF REMEDIES
GENERAL

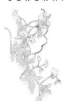

BRY.
Dry cough, worse for the least movement. Thirsty for large amounts of water.

PULS.
Weepy, wanting fuss and attention. Thirstless.

CAUST.
Hollow, dry cough; unable to produce phlegm. Sympathetic emotional state, with sensitivity to injustice. Complaints better in damp weather.

103

Phytolacca

[PHYT.]

American nightshade, or pokeroot, was used by the Native Americans to treat skin complaints and as a purgative. To prepare the remedy, the roots are dried and powdered, steeped in alcohol, then strained and filtered.

CONFIRMATION

Plant: PHYTOLACCA AMERICANA *American nightshade*

WORSE
movement

WORSE
cold weather

WORSE
night

THIRST
cold drinks

- *Glandular inflammations and swellings; hard and sensitive*
- *Rheumatic pains*
- *Sharp pains appear, disappear quickly*

RIGHT *American nightshade, or pokeroot, is used to treat glandular problems, especially mastitis.*

General indications
Useful for inflamed glands, especially mammary glands and tonsils. Glands swollen, hard, aching. Sharp pains appear and disappear suddenly. Tendons and joints sore, aching, feeling bruised. Also useful for pains in muscles and joints (as in rheumatism) particularly the neck and back. Sharp pains appear and disappear suddenly. General restlessness with a desire for motion, but the movement makes the symptoms worse.

Mental and emotional state
No marked symptoms.

Modalities
Worse: cold, damp weather; motion; night. Better: cold drinks; dry weather.

Food/drink
No marked desires or aversions.

COMPLAINTS

❖ **Sore throat**
Tonsils swollen, especially on right side. Throat appears dark red and feels hot, rough, and narrow. Pain shoots into ears when swallowing. Feeling of lump in the throat. Cannot swallow hot drinks, but better for cold drinks. Follicular tonsillitis (ulcers on tonsils).

❖ **Aches and pains**
Pains fly like electric shocks. Aching, sore, bruised feeling all over body. Person inclined to move, but movement worsens pains.

CHILDREN

❖ **Teething**
Difficult, painful; child wants to bite down on something hard, or bite gums or teeth together.

❖ **Mumps**
Swelling of parotid gland.

WOMEN

❖ **Mastitis**
Breasts hard and very sensitive. Hard lumps. Enlarged glands under arms. Pain goes all over body when breastfeeding. Mastitis during pregnancy or when breastfeeding.

❖ **Cracked nipples**
When breastfeeding. Pain in the nipple radiates all over body.

COMPARISON OF REMEDIES
FOR MASTITIS

BELL.

Similar symptoms to *Phyt.* of mastitis. Bright red discoloration of the skin and red streaks radiate from the nipples. *Bell.* is generally more red, and likely to have a fever; symptoms come on quickly and forcefully. The pains of *Bell.* are throbbing.

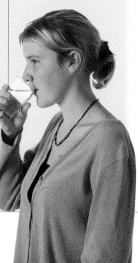

LEFT *Cold drinks may help to alleviate* Phytolacca *symptoms.*

Podophyllum

[PODO.]

The Podophyllum *homeopathic remedy was first proved in the 19th century. The root of the plant is macerated and steeped in alcohol; the mixture is then strained to prepare the tincture. It is a useful remedy for digestive problems.*

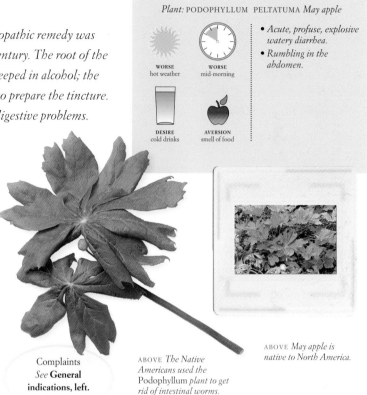

CONFIRMATION

Plant: PODOPHYLLUM PELTATUMA *May apple*

WORSE
hot weather

WORSE
mid-morning

DESIRE
cold drinks

AVERSION
smell of food

- *Acute, profuse, explosive watery diarrhea.*
- *Rumbling in the abdomen.*

ABOVE *May apple is native to North America.*

General indications
Podo. is very useful for acute diarrhea with profuse watery, explosive, and offensive stool. Feel weak and faint after passing stool. Frequent gushing or involuntary stool, sudden and painless. Cramping pain with gurgling or rumbling in the abdomen that can be heard before the stool. Loud flatus is passed with the stool. Diarrhea after drinking water. Babies with teething difficulties with this picture of diarrhea.

Mental and emotional state
No marked symptoms.

Modalities
Worse: after drinking water, eating; hot weather, mid-morning.

Food/drink
Desires: cold drinks
Aversions: smell of food

Complaints
See General
indications, left.

ABOVE *The Native Americans used the* Podophyllum *plant to get rid of intestinal worms.*

COMPARISON OF REMEDIES

DIARRHEA

ALOE
Traveler's diarrhea with lots of wind and burning pains. Often cannot pass stool without also passing urine at the same time. Sudden urge to pass stool, which is gushing and watery. Great sense of insecurity, not sure if gas or stool will come, has to hurry to the toilet after eating or drinking. Weakness and loss of power of the sphincter – "accidents" may occur in bed, without the person noticing. Also suitable for dysentery with burning pains.

CHINA
Diarrhea from eating fruit or drinking milk or beer. Stool is brown, yellow, watery, and may contain undigested food. Extreme weakness following profuse diarrhea.

SIL.
Constant but ineffectual desire for stool. Diarrhea comes on from poor eating habits, teething, hot weather, or because dry stools have remained a long time in the rectum. The diarrhea is painless but offensive, and may contain undigested food.

Pulsatilla

[PULS.]

Native to Europe, the Pulsatilla *plant has been used in herbal medicine to treat a wide range of complaints including digestive disorders and headache. The tincture is made from the whole fresh plant when in flower. Its key uses include emotional problems and women's complaints.*

General indications

Pulsatilla affects many parts of the body but primarily the mind, mucous membranes, and genitourinary organs. Discharges are thick, bland, yellow. A main characteristic is the shifting, changeable nature of both physical and emotional symptoms. Inflammations are not of a serious nature and do not progress to deep destructive lesions. Problems in pregnancy. Right side. Warm-blooded, better in the open air.

Mental and emotional state

Affectionate, mild, emotional; seeks attention, and craves sympathy and comforting. Child wants to be carried. Weeps easily. May feel unloved, left out. May alternate between gentleness and irritability, but never violent. Often worse in the evening.

Modalities

Worse: any warmth – of air, room, bed, food; fatty or rich foods.
Better: cold food and drink, cool air, open windows, cool bath; cooling off even when chilled; gentle motion.

Food/drink

Desires: cold food, alcoholic drinks, eggs, ice cream, peanut butter, many things.
Aversions: butter, eggs, fruit, meat, warm food and drink.
Thirst: none.

CONFIRMATION

Plant: PULSATILLA NIGRICANS
meadow anemone, pasque flower, wind flower

SENSATION
warm

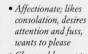

WORSE
warmth

THIRST
absent

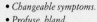

BETTER
open air

- *Affectionate; likes consolation, desires attention and fuss, wants to please*
- *Changeable symptoms.*
- *Profuse, bland, yellow/green discharges*
- *Thirstless*
- *Better for open air.*
- *Aversion to fats, rich foods*

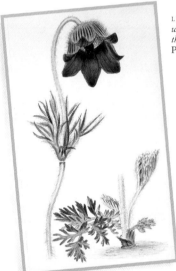

LEFT *The windflower is the source for* Pulsatilla.

COMPARISON OF REMEDIES

GENERAL

ARS.
Restless, anxious, chilly; burning pains better for warm applications.

IGN.
Ailments from emotional upset; sighing; contradictory symptoms.

KALI BIC.
Thick, sticky, ropey discharges, leaving areas raw and sore.

PHOS.
Chilly; worse for cold. Thirst for cold drinks.

COMPLAINTS

❖ **Headache**
Pain in the forehead, temples or sides, or on one side only. Constricting or bursting feeling. Heat makes the person dizzy. Feels better with a cold compress, pressure, and moving gently in the open air. Headache with indigestion caused by fatty, rich food. Generally better for bending forward, lying or sitting still, and moving the eyes.

❖ **Eye infections**
Conjunctivitis with thick, yellow, bland discharge. Suitable for children with the characteristic discharge. Sties of the upper lid that feel better for warm or cold bathing, and in the open air.

❖ **Common cold**
Frequent sneezing, yellow-green discharge that may become foul smelling and cause the nostrils to be sore and raw. Nose is more stuffed up in a warm room, feels better in the cool air.

❖ **Cough**
Dry in the evening and at night, but loose in the morning. Irritating tickle in the throat causes cough. Worse for lying down, must sit up in bed. Phlegm may be difficult to bring up, and is yellow, and sticky, with a bitter or salty taste.

❖ **Earache**
Infections, otitis media, with a stopped-up feeling or shooting pain. Extra mucus in the ears causes whistling, roaring, and ringing noises. Discharge is bland, itchy, profuse, and contains pus.

❖ **Digestive disorders**
Stomachache caused by fatty, rich food, or fruit. Mouth covered with a thick, white fur; breath bad. Nausea with a bitter, slimy, or acid taste in the mouth. Pains in the lower abdomen that move around with rumbling, gurgling noises. Particularly averse to fatty foods, such as port and milk. Nausea from the smell of smoke.

❖ **Diarrhea**
Soft stool, with slimy, green mucus. A good remedy for mucous diarrhea in childhood diseases such as measles and chicken pox.

❖ **Cystitis**
Scanty urine, with a strong ammoniac smell. Burning pain, during and after urination, at the opening of the urethra. Bland, yellow-green discharge.

❖ **Fever**
Chilliness without thirst. Although chilly, the open or cool air is preferred. Heat is intolerable; uncovers.

❖ **Aches and pains**
Pains in limbs shift rapidly; worse for warmth. Swelling moves around; first one joint is swollen, then another.

CHILDREN

❖ **Measles**
With characteristic mental, general, skin, and catarrhal symptoms.

❖ **Mumps**
With metastasis (spreading) to breasts and testes.

WOMEN

❖ **Nausea in pregnancy**
With aversion to all food (*see above Digestive disorders*); vomiting mucus in the morning.

❖ **Childbirth**
Suffocating and fainting spells, must have doors or windows open during labor. Labor pains not strong enough, irregular, changeable. Abnormal presentation (*Pulsatilla* may enable the baby to turn around if presenting breech).

❖ **Breastfeeding**
Promotes the flow of milk, if insufficient.

MEN

❖ **Nonspecific urethritis**
NSU or prostate inflammation, with urinary symptoms (*see Cystitis*), and thick yellow discharge from urethra.

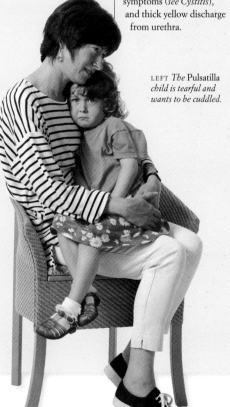

LEFT *The* Pulsatilla *child is tearful and wants to be cuddled.*

107

Rhus toxicodendron

[RHUS T.]

Commonly known as poison ivy, this plant can cause a violent skin reaction in some people. The homeopathic tincture is made from the fresh leaves, picked during the night when they are at their most poisonous. It is used as a remedy for skin complaints and joint pain.

CONFIRMATION

Plant: RHUS TOXICODENDRON
poison oak, poison ivy, sumach, swamp dogwood

WORSE cold damp weather

WORSE cold drinks

BETTER heat

BETTER continued movement

- *Extreme restlessness, physical and emotional*
- *Worse at night*
- *Strains and sprains from injuries to joints, overstretching, overlifting; worse for rest, first movement, better for continued movement*
- *Worse for cold and damp; better for warmth*

General indications
Affections of the skin: red eruptions, swelling just underneath the skin, vesicles, with intense itching. Joint pains from injuries or overuse. Extreme restlessness; person cannot find a comfortable place to rest, tosses and turns. Symptoms are worse at night and are made worse or brought on by exposure to cold and damp. Great thirst.

Better: continued motion, moving affected parts; change of position; heat (warm wraps, bath, warm dry weather, warm drinks).

Food/drink
Desires: milk, cold drinks, tonics, candy. **Aversions:** alcoholic stimulants; food, after eating a little. **Thirst:** intense.

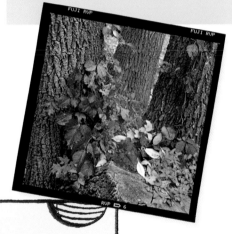
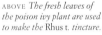

ABOVE *The fresh leaves of the poison ivy plant are used to make the* Rhus t. *tincture.*

Mental and emotional state
Sad, wants to be alone. Restlessness appears in the mind as well, so the person is impatient and fretful, anxious,"itching to get out."

Modalities
Worse: exposure to wet, cold air or draft when hot or sweaty; beginning motion; sprains; rest; after midnight; cold drinks, cold food.

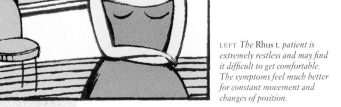

LEFT *The* Rhus t. *patient is extremely restless and may find it difficult to get comfortable. The symptoms feel much better for constant movement and changes of position.*

COMPLAINTS

❖ **Emotional problems**
Very restless, irritable. Anxious when indoors, in bed. Tosses and turns. Nervous restlessness will drive person out of bed.

❖ **Headache**
Head hot and heavy, brain feels loose. Painful to touch. Stupefying headache; must lie down. Headache after cold bath, wetting the hair, in wet weather.

❖ **Eye affections**
Pain behind the eyes, worse for motion. Inflammation and swelling of eyes. Sties. In newborn infants, swelling of the eyelids from exposure to cold and damp.

❖ **Earache**
Otitis media, inflamed internally and externally, with throat swollen and sore. Discharges of bloody pus. Swelling of glands behind the ears.

❖ **Common cold**
Colds with violent sneezing and runny nose in the morning. Throat swollen, causing difficulty in swallowing. Glands swollen and hard, with dry mouth and unquenchable thirst, but worse for cold drinks and swallowing. Voice is hoarse, strained from overuse but improves on continued use. Tongue coated, except for triangular red tip.

❖ **Influenza**
Aching, shooting pains in joints and bones, with heaviness, stiffness. Person feels sore, bruised, exhausted. Painful at first movement, but improves on continued motion.

❖ **Skin rash**
Urticaria, hives with burning itching rash, worse for scratching. Itching and restlessness; sleep disturbed on account of the eruptions.

❖ **Joint pain, injuries**
Hot painful swelling of joints. Tearing pains in ligaments, tendons, and muscles. Limbs feel stiff and paralyzed. Sciatica. Complaints from sports/exercise injuries overstretching, overlifting. Rheumatism, joint pain from strains or sprains; worse for first movement, better on continued movement.

CHILDREN

❖ **Chicken pox, measles**
Where rash is intensely burning and itching; better for hot water. (*See above Eye affections.*)

WOMEN

❖ **Threatened abortion**
From overlifting and overstraining muscles and ligaments.

MEN

❖ **Testes**
Metastasis of mumps to testes. Scrotum dark red, swollen, with intense itching.

❖ **Prostate**
Pain in prostate when urging to pass stool.

LEFT *One of the main uses of the* Rhus t. *remedy is the treatment of pain in the joints, including rheumatism.*

APIS
Skin swollen, bright shiny red; worse for warmth.

BELL.
Redness of skin with inflammations; affects blood vessels.

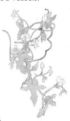

BRY.
Worse for any movement at all. Irritable, fretful, peevish; dreams of business.

RUTA
Affects periosteum, ligaments, connective tissue; worse for motion of affected part.

109

Ruta graveolens

[RUTA]

Rue has a long history of use as a herbal remedy. During the Middle Ages it was used against the plague, and it has also been used as an antidote to poison. The whole plant is gathered before flowering, then macerated and soaked in alcohol to make the tincture. It is used to treat bruised muscles and bones.

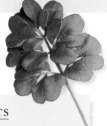

CONFIRMATION

Plant: RUTA GRAVEOLENS *common rue*

BETTER
gentle movement

BETTER
warmth

WORSE
cold air

WORSE
wind

- Sore, bruised, aching feeling
- Injuries to tendons, ligaments, periosteum
- Affected parts are worse for movement
- Worse for cold; better for warmth

LEFT *Known as the herb of grace, rue is the source for* Ruta graveolens.

General indications
Ruta graveolens **acts on fibrous tissue, ligaments, cartilage, and bones, especially joints, in cases of trauma and overexertion. Parts feel bruised, sore, aching, tender.**

Mental and emotional state
Dissatisfied with self, disposed to weep. Imagines deception.

Modalities
Worse: overexertion; cold air, wind, damp, wet; lying, sitting, stooping; raw foods. Better: continued gentle movement; warmth; daytime.

Food/drink
No marked desires or aversions.

COMPLAINTS

❖ **Eyestrain**
Eyes feel red, hot, with aching and burning sensations; vision is blurred. Useful after long periods of close work. Better in open air; worse for warmth

❖ **Injuries, aches, and pains**
Bruised, aching, lame feeling in tendons, ligaments, muscle sheaths. Bruises to periosteum. Back pain, better for lying on the back. Nodules on the periosteum and tendons after injury. Bruises go away slowly and leave a hardened spot, with thickening of the bone. Lameness after sprains, especially of

wrists and ankles. Fibrous growths on tendons from overuse of hands or other parts (repetitive strain injury). Area surrounding joint feels weak; the pain is more noticeable when joint is in use . First movement after rest is painful, then pain eases after gentle movement. *Ruta* is given after *Arnica* and *Rhus toxicodendron* when the injury is not healing. Inflammations around small joints, such as wrist, knee, ankle.

WOMEN

❖ **Rectal prolapse**
After childbirth, from strained pelvic floor muscles.

COMPARISON OF REMEDIES

FOR INJURY TO JOINTS

ARN.
Initial bruises, worse for touch. Sore bruised sensation all over body.

BRY.
Strains, sprains worse with every movement.

RHUS T.
Joint pains worse during initial movement after rest, but improve on continued movement. Muscles and tendons affected.

Sepia
[SEP.]

Hahnemann proved the Sepia *remedy on observing that the symptoms in an artist improved after he had been licking his brushes which were soaked with sepia paint. The remedy is made from the pigment of cuttlefish ink. It is a good remedy for women's complaints.*

CONFIRMATION

Animal: SEPIA OFFICINALIS *cuttlefish*

SENSATION
chilly

WORSE
cold

BETTER
gentle movement

BETTER
warmth

- *Ailments after hormonal changes*
- *Chilly*
- *Uncommunicative*
- *Worse for consolation*
- *Better for vigorous exercise and dancing*
- *Dragging pains*

COMPLAINTS

General indications
Venous circulation and female pelvic organs are affected. Symptoms are predominantly left-sided. Sensitive to extremes of hot and cold. Sepia affects digestion. Ailments relating to hormonal changes.

Mental and emotional state
Looks after other people and then becomes exhausted, stops caring, and loses interest. Wants to be left alone; hates fuss; can become angry.

Modalities
Worse: cold; pregnancy, menopause, sexual excesses, abortion. Better: vigorous exercise, warmth; when busy.

Food/drink
Desires: alcoholic drinks, cold drinks, chocolate, pickles, candy, sour foods.

❖ **Headache**
Pain bursting, shooting, pressing, throbbing, in waves.

❖ **Cough**
Hacking, irritating, loose; disturbs sleep. Copious, yellow-white mucus with salty taste.

❖ **Digestive disorders**
Morning nausea; nausea at smell, sight, or thought of food. Nausea after eating, or relieved by eating; food and bile vomited in the morning. Empty sensation in stomach, only relieved temporarily by eating. Ravenously hungry or easily satisfied; cravings.

❖ **Constipation**
Person strains to expel a hard stool. Pain precedes passing of stool.

WOMEN

❖ **Hemorrhoids**
During pregnancy.

❖ **Nausea, vomiting, constipation**
During pregnancy (*see* above *Digestive disorders*).

❖ **Labor pains**
Dragging sensation in the lower part of the uterus as if everything would fall out. Retained placenta.

❖ **Postnatal trauma**
To pelvic floor; pelvic organs relaxed. Prolapse.

❖ **Urinary problems**
Caused by laxity of pelvic floor muscles. Urine leaks on coughing or laughing. Constant urge to urinate; urine is milky, burning, bloody.

COMPARISON OF REMEDIES

GENERAL

LACH.
Hot person, worse for heat; expressive; wounds bleed freely.

NAT-M.
Thirsty person, worse for heat of sun and for exertion; craves salt.

PHOS.
Desires company, fearful; likes cold drinks; exhaustion worse for exertion.

LEFT *The cuttlefish, the source for* Sepia, *is found mainly in the Mediterranean Sea.*

Silica

[SIL.]

Silica is prepared from silicon dioxide, found in quartz, flint, and sandstone. The homeopathic remedy is prepared by trituration with lactose sugar. It helps expel foreign bodies, such as splinters and thorns.

CONFIRMATION

Mineral: SILICON DIOXIDE *quartz, rock crystal, pure flint*

SENSATION
chilly

WORSE
cold

BETTER
warmth

THIRST
cold drinks

- *Chilly – worse for cold, better for warmth*
- *Sensitive, yielding, mild, but with inner resistance*
- *Easy perspiration and suppuration*
- *Promotes expulsion of foreign bodies in tissues*
- *Ill effects of vaccination*

General indications

Glandular affections, abscesses. Promotes the expulsion of splinters, thorns, and other foreign matter from the body. Boils are slow to develop. Ill effects of vaccination. Delicate, yielding, timid type of person, though with inner resistance. Extremely chilly; cannot get warm even with exercise. Perspires easily, especially head and feet (often with smelly feet). Lacks stamina.

Mental and emotional state

Sensitive, easily startled, anxious, fearful, self-doubting. Yielding nature, but has stronger inner core (can be obstinate, with fixed ideas). Appearance is very important. Overworked mental state.

Modalities

Worse: cold (air, drafts, damp, uncovering, bathing); after vaccination; milk. Better: warm (especially warm wraps to the head), warm room; profuse urination.

Food/drink

Desires: cold food, milk. Thirsty. Aversions: meat, mother's milk.

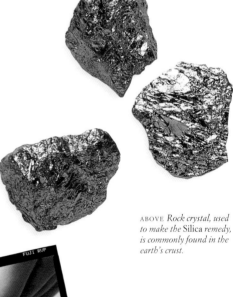

ABOVE *Rock crystal, used to make the* Silica *remedy, is commonly found in the earth's crust.*

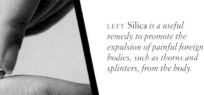

LEFT Silica *is a useful remedy to promote the expulsion of painful foreign bodies, such as thorns and splinters, from the body.*

COMPLAINTS

❖ Headache
From fasting, not eating at the correct time. Headache characterized by modalities: worse for mental effort, noise, jarring, movement, light, bending forward, cold, any draft of air. Better for warmth applied to head, warmth generally, wrapping head tightly. Profuse sweat on head. Vision is worse after headache.

❖ Tooth abscesses
Abscess at root of teeth, foul pus discharges, worse for cold water. Offensive odor.

❖ Earache
Roaring in the ears. Perforated eardrum; bloody, smelly, thick discharge. Blocked feeling and itchy inside the ear, better for yawning or swallowing.

❖ Constipation
Constant desire to pass stool, but effort is ineffectual. Stool hard, dry, light colored, but difficult to pass. The stool may be partly passed but then slip back into the rectum; the person becomes tired, gives up, and the stool recedes.

❖ Diarrhea
From poor eating habits, teething, hot weather, or because dry stools have been a long time in the rectum. Diarrhea is offensive, painless, and contains undigested food.

BELOW Silica *is a useful remedy for ear infections when accompanied by typical* Silica *general and mental symptoms.*

❖ Skin wounds
Every little injury becomes inflamed, festers. Skin wounds slow to heal, with easy suppuration: abcesses, boils, ulcers, pustules. Itching, worse at night, better for warm application. Silica promotes expulsion of foreign bodies such as thorns or splinters from tissues.

WOMEN

❖ Mastitis
Hard lumps in the breast; sudden, sharp pain during breastfeeding.

❖ Sore nipples
Sore nipples ulcerate easily. Darting, burning pains in left nipple.

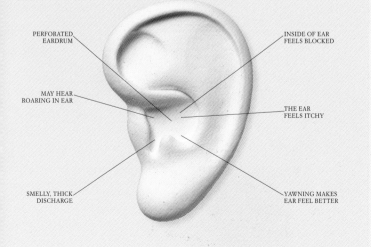

PERFORATED EARDRUM

MAY HEAR ROARING IN EAR

SMELLY, THICK DISCHARGE

INSIDE OF EAR FEELS BLOCKED

THE EAR FEELS ITCHY

YAWNING MAKES EAR FEEL BETTER

COMPARISON OF REMEDIES

GENERAL

CALC.
Chilly, sweaty on head at night. Sour-smelling diarrhea with teething difficulties of babies and children.

HEP.
Ultrasensitive to pain, cold, slightest draft. Deep abscesses of teeth, skin, glands; swollen with extreme pain. Formation of pus that has not yet begun to discharge. Intolerant of slightest touch.

MERC.
Increased secretions: saliva, sweat, etc. Profuse green discharges that burn or sting. Foul odors, more offensive than *Hep.* or *Sil.* Sensitive to changes of temperature – worse from cold or heat.

PULS.
Bland, yellow/green discharges with many complaints. Warm person, craving open air or open windows, usually thirstless. Emotional state is gentle and tearful while seeking attention and sympathy.

Spongia tosta
[SPONG.]

Proved by Hahnemann himself, the Spongia *remedy is made from the sea sponge. The sponge is roasted brown, then steeped in alcohol. The liquid is strained and filtered to make the homeopathic tincture. It is an excellent remedy for croup.*

General indications
Main parts of the body affected are the larynx and the trachea. Extreme dryness of mucous membranes. Useful in cases of cough, croup, and sore throat. Waking from sleep in suffocation, and state of anxiety. Difficulty breathing. Great dryness of all air passages. Sensation of "breathing through a dry sponge." Symptoms become worse during sleep.

BELOW *Smoking will aggravate the condition of the* Spongia *patient.*

Mental and emotional state
Wakes at night with great fear. Starting from sleep.

Modalities
Worse: tobacco, fats; cold, dry wind; lying with head low. Better: swallowing warm drinks.

Food/drink
No marked desires or aversions. Excessive thirst, great hunger.

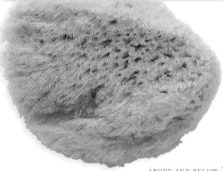

ABOVE AND BELOW *The sea sponge from the Mediterranean and other seas is used to prepare* Spongia tosta.

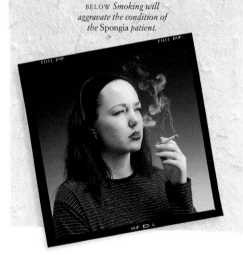

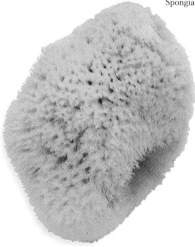

COMPLAINTS

❖ Cough

Dry, constant, barking, hollow, sawing, crowing. Disturbs sleep; on waking there is burning in chest and throat. Burning, sore, bruised pain in the chest. Better for warm drinks. Cough is worse in a warm room, and for talking.

❖ Croup

Cough dry, painful, rasping; sound begins with tickling low down in the chest, or feeling that there is something blocking the larynx. No mucus, no rattle, no expectoration. After much difficult breathing and coughing a little sputum comes up, but only as far as the throat. Acute anxiety with cough; when waking in the night there is a feeling of suffocation. Worse for inspiration, and before midnight. *Spongia* given if *Aconite* fails.

❖ Laryngitis

Larynx inflamed. Dry, burning, constricted, painful; worse for touch, talking, or swallowing. Hoarseness. Worse for turning the head, or for sweet food or drinks, which tickle the throat.

BELOW Spongia tosta *symptoms include difficult breathing and a dry, painful cough.*

VERY DRY, INFLAMED THROAT

SENSE OF BURNING IN CHEST

COMPARISON OF REMEDIES

COUGH/CROUP

ACON.

When symptoms come on suddenly, after person has been in a cold, dry wind. Thirsty for cold drinks. (*Spong.* follows *Acon.* well, or is indicated if *Acon.* does not relieve symptoms.)

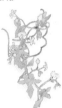

ANT-T.

Much rattling of mucus in chest, but with no energy to expel it.

BRY.

Painful, dry hacking cough from irritation in the throat. Must sit up to cough. Worse after eating and drinking, vomiting, or for any movement. Stitches in chest.

CAUST.

Hollow hard, dry cough. raw soreness of chest. Difficult to bring anything up; must be swallowed. Better for drinking cold water. Often with pain in the hips.

DROS.

Dry irritating cough, with fits of deep barking, or choking, prolonged and incessant. Can hardly breathe. Worse at night. Violent tickle in the throat, as if from a feather. Deep, hoarse voice.

HEP.

For later stages of croup, where person is chilly, and oversensitive to any external impression: sound, light, touch. Better for heat.

PHOS.

Hard, dry, tight cough that may be violent, exhausting, or cause trembling. Sensation as if there is a weight on the chest. Coughs up lots of phlegm, which may be salty, yellow, or bloodstreaked. Desires cold iced drinks.

Staphysagria

[STAPH.]

The ancient Greeks and Romans used this plant as an emetic and purgative. To make the remedy, the seeds are dried, ground, and steeped in alcohol; the mixture is then filtered and strained to make the tincture.

CONFIRMATION

Plant: DELPHINIUM STAPHYSAGRIA *licebane*

WORSE
negative emotions

WORSE
touch

WORSE
cold

BETTER
warmth

- Ailments from suppressed emotions: anger, indignation, insults
- Great sensitivity to touch
- Cystitis after coitus, catheterization
- After surgical incisions, clean-cut wounds, stab wounds, cesarian

General indications
Emotions are aroused in anger or indignation. Extreme sensitivity to the least unpleasant impression – in particular cannot bear any criticism and takes offense when none is meant, becoming indignant at slight offense or rudeness, and angry if opposed. Functional disorders such as headache, pain in some part, colic can be brought on after this kind of emotional incident. An important remedy for particular kinds of mental and physical wounds. Acts on urinary and pelvic organs. Pains from injury from sharp cutting instruments, or from stretching sphincters, e.g. childbirth. Pains worse for touch or pressure.

Mental and emotional state
Symptoms relate to, or are caused by, feelings of indignation: "Why me?" "What have I done?" Feeling injured but suppressing feelings of anger or hurt.

After love disappointment, or feelings of being humiliated, hurt, or insulted, real or imagined. May rationalize to oneself, but deep down feels injured. *Staphysagria* **may also be appropriate for a person who feels wrongly punished, or who is the victim of bullying or mugging and dwells on the incident, has no recourse; cannot do anything about it; sense of injustice prominent.**

Modalities
Worse: emotions (chagrin, vexation, indignation), quarrels; touch; cold, cold drinks. Better: warmth; rest; breakfast.

Food/drink
Desires: soup, candy, alcoholic drinks, meat. Aversions: milk, cheese, solid foods.

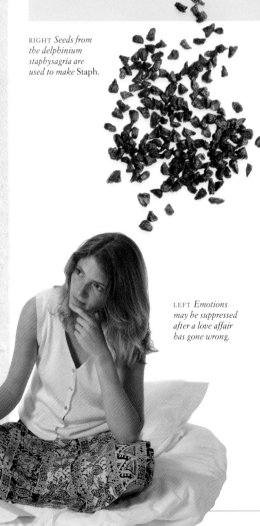

RIGHT *Seeds from the delphinium staphysagria are used to make* Staph.

LEFT *Emotions may be suppressed after a love affair has gone wrong.*

COMPLAINTS

❖ **Digestive disorders**
Colic and diarrhea, or any stomach problems associated with the emotional states described above. Sea sickness with dizziness, vertigo. Take *Staphysagria* for nausea, or travel sickness, with accompanying sense of indignation as described above.

❖ **Cystitis**
Pain when not urinating distinguishes this from other cystitis remedies. Sensation of pressure upon the bladder, feels as if it did not empty. Burning during urination. Copious and involuntary urination, especially on coughing.

WOMEN

❖ **Cystitis**
From oversensitivity of bladder, so that cystitis follows coitus.

❖ **Childbirth**
Urinary difficulties, pelvic pains, pain and/or infection of wounds after operations to sexual organs e.g. episiotomy, cesarian, abortion, etc. with the emotional state of *Staph.* These feelings of anger or humiliation may arise from an experience of childbirth when more procedures

BELOW Staphysagria is a good remedy for urinary problems in both men and women.

were carried out than expected. Even though the woman appears to accept the circumstances, suppressing her own feelings, inside she may feel she has been interfered with, to the point of violation.

MEN

❖ **Prostatitis**
Frequent urination; burning in urethra when not urinating. Pains extend from anus to urethra.

❖ **Orchitis**
From mumps.

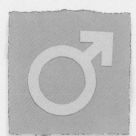

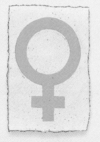

SPECIAL APPLICATIONS
Post surgery: pain after surgical incisions, clean-cut wounds, stab wounds; episiotomy, cesarian, laparoscopy, etc.

SPECIAL APPLICATIONS
As its common name, Licebane, suggests, this plant is known for its use in treating lice. The *Staph.* tincture can be used on head lice and nits, pubic hair lice (crabs). Wash hair in 0.6 fl.oz. (15ml) of tincture. Do not rinse out: leave on for at least two hours, but preferably overnight. Repeat process in two weeks to prevent reinfestation.

COMPARISON OF REMEDIES

GENERAL

BELL-P.
Trauma of internal or pelvic organs, either from injury or surgery. Wounds are extremely sore, cannot be touched. Generally worse for any form of cold.

CHAM.
Anger is openly expressed. Wants many things, rejects them when offered them. Screams from intense unbearable pains.

IGN.
Worse for emotions of grief, with sighing; consolation aggravates. Changing states of mind.

SEP.
Emotional indifference. Hormonal imbalances cause problems.

Sulfur

[SUL.]

Sulfur has the most symptoms of any remedy in the Materia Medica because it has been so extensively proved and has a long history of use in medicine. It is prepared either by triturating the flowers of sulfur with lactose sugar or by dissolving them in alcohol to form a tincture.

CONFIRMATION

Mineral: SULFUR *brimstone, flowers of sulfur*

SENSATION
warm

WORSE
11 a.m.

BETTER
warm, dry weather

BETTER
open air

- *Complaints slow to improve*
- *Warm; wants air, wants windows open*
- *Burning pains and sensations*
- *Redness of parts*
- *Desires sweets and spicy food*
- *Offensive discharges*

General indications

Burning and/or itching sensations, of any part of the body, worse for warmth of bed. Red lips, face, eyelids, orifices, skin. Warm people who have a desire for open air, cannot stand warm or close rooms, and become very hot in bed. May become very weak from not eating. Strong desires for candy and spicy food. Offensive odors from secretions: perspiration, stool, urine, foot sweat. Tendency to appear unclean or untidy. Dislikes bathing, which often makes complaints worse. Complaints are worse, or come on, at night, or late morning around 11 a.m.

Mental and emotional state

The remedy picture is so broad that it could belong to any kind of person. However, the typical *Sulfur* state of mind is dominated by the imagination. **Person may dwell on religious or philosophical subjects; a more practical** *Sulfur* **person will also be creative and idealistic. Therefore they may be untidy, or disinclined to be concerned with the physical needs of the body; they may dislike washing and bathing and appear lazy and indifferent to personal appearance. They may make many plans but seldom carry them out.**

Modalities

Worse: bathing; becoming heated, warm or close room; early morning, 11 a.m., night. Better: open air; motion; dry, warm weather.

Food/drink

Desires: fatty foods and candy, highly seasoned food, alcoholic drinks, meat. Aversions: eggs, meat, olives, strong cheese.

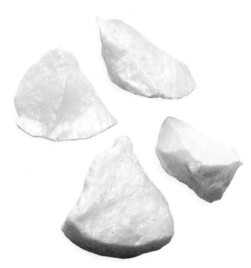

ABOVE *A yellow powder is extracted from the mineral known as Flowers of Sulfur.*

CAUTION

Almost every remedy will have some comparison with *Sulfur*. Review symptoms carefully before deciding.

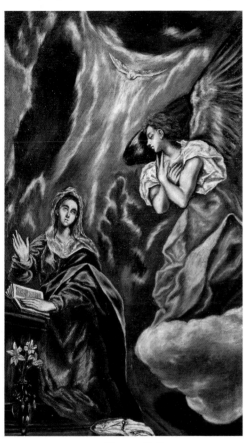

ABOVE *The mental* Sulfur
picture often includes deep
intellectual and theological
speculation.

COMPLAINTS

❖ **Headache**
Feels as if wearing
"tight hat." Burning
sensations: top of head,
soles of feet, anywhere.
With nausea. Worse for
eating, bending forward,
and in early morning;
better for coolness or
cold compresses.
Headache caused by
indigestion, overeating.

❖ **Eye affections**
Inflammation with
burning, heat, redness.
Eyes feel gritty. Eyelids
red, itchy during the day;
glued together in the
morning. Cannot stand
washing eyes.

❖ **Common cold**
Brought on by bathing,
overexertion, overheating,
or becoming cold. Much
sneezing. Watery trickle of
acrid, burning discharge
from nose. After *Aconite*.

❖ **Influenza**
Very sensitive to open air,
drafts. Burning pains or
sensations: top of head,
chest, feet. After *Aconite*.

❖ **Cough**
Disturbs sleep. Dry at
night, loose during the
day. Chest congested.
Wants fresh air.

❖ **Indigestion, colic**
Abdomen distended with
wind, noise of grumbling
in bowel. Extremely
urgent diarrhea in early
morning. Burning pains in
stomach. Extremely
hungry around 11 a.m.

CHILDREN

❖ **Diarrhea**
Diarrhea during teething.
Redness around anus, lips,
eyelids. Stool acrid,
irritating, and causes red,
inflamed diaper rash.
Rough skin, hair. Feels hot
at night; throws covers off.

❖ **Childhood diseases**
Itching in last stages of
chicken pox, measles,
mumps, or other
symptoms worse for
warmth and/or bathing.

COMPARISON OF REMEDIES

GENERAL

ACON.
Inflammations in the early
stages of illness.

NUX V.
Similar stomach/digestive
symptoms, but usually
more chilly.

ACUTE ILLNESSES
Sulfur can be used in the later
stages of acute illnesses, after other
remedies have helped in the early
stages. In each case refer to
general characteristics.

Symphytum

[SYMPH.]

This homeopathic remedy is prepared from the comfrey plant. Long known to herbalists for its healing properties, the comfrey plant is used to aid the mending of broken bones. To prepare the remedy, the fresh root is chopped and steeped in alcohol, and the mixture is then strained and filtered to make the tincture.

CONFIRMATION

Plant: SYMPHYTUM GENUS *comfrey, knitbone, boneset, bruisewort, blackwort, gumplant, healing plant.*

BETTER
warmth

BETTER
gentle movement

WORSE
touch

WORSE
pressure

- *Injuries to bones, periosteum, cartilage*
- *Blows from blunt instruments*
- *Better for gentle motion, warmth*
- *Worse for touch, motion, pressure*

General indications
As the common names for the plant suggest, this remedy has been known for a long time to promote the healing of wounds, particularly injuries to bones, cartilage, and periosteum. It is also the main remedy for pain in the eyeball, from trauma or injury.

Mental and emotional state
No marked symptoms.

Modalities
**Worse: touch, motion, pressure.
Better: warmth; gentle motion.**

Food/drink
No marked desires or aversions.

COMPLAINTS

❖ **Eye injury**
This remedy is specifically indicated for traumatic injury to the eyeball or surrounding bones. Give after *Arnica*, which reduces the initial swelling.

❖ **Fractures**
Broken bones; damage to cartilage; damage to periosteum, especially where bones are close to the surface, e.g. shins. Fractures and broken bones that are slow to heal.

BELOW *The* Symphytum *remedy is prepared from the comfrey plant.*

COMPARISON OF REMEDIES

GENERAL

ARN.
Sore, bruised feeling. First stages of sprains and strains. Other remedies may be indicated after the initial trauma is better. *Arn.* will accelerate repair of bruises or other damaged tissues, and help to reduce inflammations.

RHUS T.
Strains, sprains, muscular problems, stiff and painful on the first movement but relieved by motion.

CAUTION
Always judge the seriousness of any injury and use homeopathic remedies in conjunction with other commonsense measures to promote healing, such as rest, elevation, the use of ice packs, immobilization. Seek medical attention if necessary.

RUTA
Injury to soft tissue: cartilage. ligaments, joints. Blows to the eyeball. *Ruta* more for tissues closer to the bone.

HYP.
Injury to nerve, nerve-rich tissue: falling on spine, blows to spine or head, crushing tips of fingers or toes. Injuries from puncture wounds and shooting pains

LED.
Puncture wounds as from nails. Parts become swollen, with mottled appearance, feels cold to touch is better for cold applications.

CAUTION
Before using the remedy it is necessary that any resetting of bones takes place, since once the remedy is taken the bones will heal very quickly and strongly.

Urtica urens

[URT-U.]

The stinging nettle provides the source for
Urtica urens. *The fresh plant, picked when in*
flower, is chopped and then steeped in alcohol;
the mixture is then strained and filtered to make
the tincture. It is used to treat burns, insect
bites, and urticaria.

General indications
**Allergic skin reactions,
with burning, itching,
and swelling. First-
degree burns, with
intense itching.
Scanty breast milk,
vulval itching.**

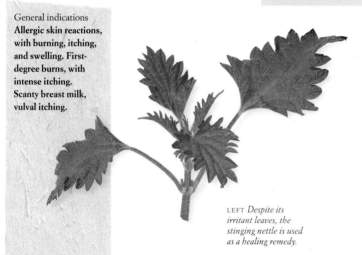

LEFT *Despite its
irritant leaves, the
stinging nettle is used
as a healing remedy.*

Mental and
emotional state
No marked symptoms.

Modalities
**Worse: cool air, cool
bathing; insect stings;
eating shellfish.
Better: rubbing.**

Food/drink
**No marked desires
or aversions, though
hives develop after
eating shellfish.**

COMPLAINTS

❖ **Skin affections**
Urticaria caused by stings
of insects or eating
shellfish. Itching blotches.
Affected area larger than
the spot where the sting
occurred. Worse for
bathing, vigorous
exercise, warmth. First-
degree burns, sunburn, or
scalds with itchiness. Use
topically as well as taking
the internal remedy.

WOMEN

❖ **Breastfeeding**
Milk absent without
apparent cause.
For stimulation of milk
production, take internally.

COMPARISON
OF REMEDIES

SKIN
CONDITIONS

APIS
Insect bites where
affected skin is hot and
worse for heat; raised, red,
shiny, flat eruptions.

CAL.
Used topically to promote
accelerated growth of
new skin; cuts, grazes, open
and damaged skin (not as
well indicated for hives
or other skin allergies).

CANTH.
Second-degree burns with
violent pains. Burns before
blisters form. Burns with
rawness and smarting.

CAUST.
Third-degree burns, scalds or
chemical burns. Burning pain,
with blisters. Ill effects from
burns; old burns that do not
heal properly.

RHUS T.
Urticaria, hives, rash, with
burning and itching. Very
restless, worse for cold,
damp, scratching.

Veratrum album

[VERAT.]

Veratrum album is made from the fresh roots of the white hellebore. It has been used as a medicinal remedy since ancient times for mania, melancholy, and epilepsy. An extremely poisonous plant, it was used by the Romans to poison arrow tips. It is given homeopathically to persons in a state of collapse.

CONFIRMATION

Plant: VERATRUM ALBUM *white hellebore*

ONSET
sudden

SENSATION
chilly

THIRST
icy drinks

BETTER
open air

- *Sudden, violent onset*
- *Icy-cold surface*
- *Cold sweat*
- *Severe vomiting and diarrhea, causing exhaustion*

General indications
A picture of collapse; extremely cold, blue, weak. Sudden and forceful onset. Severe disturbance of the gastro-intestinal tract, with simultaneous vomiting and diarrhea, ice-cold chilliness, profuse cold sweat, intense thirst, sudden weakness. Fainting.

BELOW *A* Verat. *person desires acid fruits which worsen their condition.*

Mental and emotional state
Restless, distressed. Or silent, withdrawn, sullen.

Modalities
Worse: cold drinks, fruit. Better: warm food, hot drinks, milk.

Food/drink
Desires: acid fruit, salty food, cold drinks, fruit, ice.
Aversions: warm or hot food.
Thirst: extreme, for large quantities of ice-cold water.

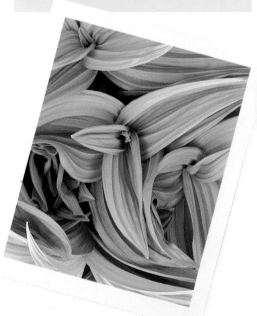

ABOVE *The white hellebore grows in the mountainous regions of Europe.*

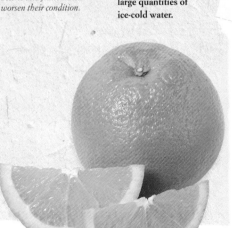

COMPLAINTS

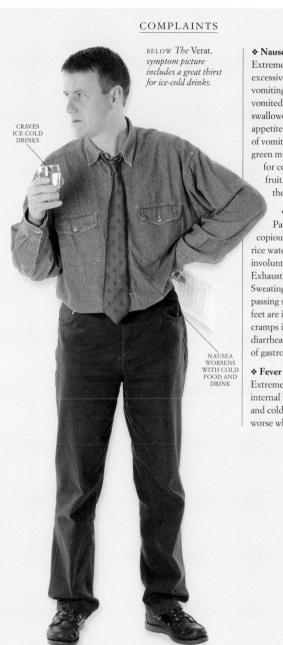

BELOW *The* Verat. *symptom picture includes a great thirst for ice-cold drinks.*

CRAVES
ICE-COLD
DRINKS

NAUSEA
WORSENS
WITH COLD
FOOD AND
DRINK

❖ **Nausea, vomiting**
Extreme nausea, excessive and violent vomiting. Cold water is vomited as soon as it is swallowed. Hunger and appetite in between bouts of vomiting. Vomiting of green mucus. Cravings for cold things and fruit, which worsen the condition.

❖ **Diarrhea**
Painful, watery, copious, greenish; like rice water; forcefully or involuntarily evacuated. Exhaustion from diarrhea. Sweating during and after passing stool. Hands and feet are icy cold. Muscle cramps in limbs during diarrhea. Symptoms of gastroenteritis.

❖ **Fever**
Extreme cold and thirst; internal heat. Skin pale and cold to touch. Feels worse while sweating.

COMPARISON OF REMEDIES

WEAKNESS / COLLAPSE

CARB-V.
Another chilly person, with very low vitality, but despite being weak and cold (even to the point where parts of the body are bluish) this person must have air, and wants to be fanned. The diarrhea is painful, also with burning in the rectum (like *Ars.*) but the stool is putrid and offensive, and even soft stool passes with difficulty. There is also wind in the digestive tract, and there is relief from belching. This situation may arise after overeating, or overindulgence in rich foods.

ARS.
A specific remedy for food poisoning. This person feels very chilly. The diarrhea produces burning pains in the stomach, bowels, rectum that feel better for heat. The burning discharges are quite thin and scanty, not profuse. The person, though restless, feels quite anxious and exhausted – almost out of proportion to the illness. There is a desire to sip at cold drinks to alleviate a burning thirst.

Guide to Using the Repertory Index

HOMEOPATHS *use a medical repertory as a reference tool to find a well-indicated remedy. The repertory systematically organizes the symptoms to be treated, and lists the remedies, in their abbreviated form, to consider for each one. Each listing is called a "rubric." The repertory in this book has a selected number of important rubrics to be used for home prescribing. These include first aid, minor injuries, acute ailments, and childbirth. (For serious conditions consult a professionally qualified homoeopath or other medical practitioner.) Although this is a limited repertory, using it will help you to understand how to use other more detailed homeopathic medical repertory books.*

In this repertory, the main rubric is followed by any subrubrics. For example if you have a cough, look up cough in the Repertory Index. This will be followed by any subrubrics, for example, dry or loose.

Naming a disease is a convenient way of talking about a collection of symptoms that sufferers have in common. Homeopaths observe the distinguishing characteristics particular to each individual in each case. Think about what the actual symptoms are. For example, a cold may include: headache, blocked or runny nose, sore throat, etc. Try to be as precise as possible.

If there is pain look up "Pain" and the description of what kind of pain it is – such as burning or throbbing, for example.

Modalities are those factors that make the person or the symptom better or worse. You should check both the general modalities and the specific symptom.

Discharges can exude from any orifice: eyes, nose, ears, mouth, vagina, penis, anus, pores (cuts, boils). However, it is the characteristics of the discharge – its color, viscosity, smell, painfulness, and so on – rather than its site, that is most helpful in determining a suitable remedy. For example, under Discharges, in the Repertory Index, it can be seen that *Pulsatilla* is applicable to green discharges whether they are from eyes, ears, or nose; *Arsenicum* is similarly applicable where discharge is also burning and acrid, whether from nose or anus; *Mercury* may have a combination of the two.

Use the symptoms in the Repertory to guide you to a selection of well-indicated remedies, then read the full description of the remedies in the Materia Medica to confirm your best choice. Remember that the remedy can be used for a number of different complaints. Ensure that the general characteristics, as well as the symptoms of the complaint, match the illness.

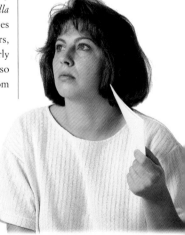

BELOW *Look up your main symptoms in the Repertory Index, for example, fever.*

FINDING THE CORRECT REMEDY

Perspiration: *Calc., Merc., Sil., Verat.*
    absent during fever: *Ars., Bell., Bry., Gels.*
    cold: *Ant-t., Ars., Carb-v., China, Cocc., Hep., Ip., Lyc., Merc., Sep., Verat.*
    hot: *Acon., Cham., Ign., Ip., Nux v., Sep.*
    profuse: *Ant-t., Ars., Calc., Carb-v., China, Hep., Lyc., Merc., Phos., Sep., Sil., Sul., Verat.*

The main rubric – in this case perspiration – is given in bold. All the remedies that follow this main rubric are characteristically and generally sweaty.

- The subrubrics define the main one, and they are therefore indented after it. In our example, "absent during fever" is a subrubric of perspiration, so the remedies that follow it are indicated for a fever without sweat.
- The remedies in the subrubrics "cold" and "hot" tell you about the person's body heat during a sweat. Although *Arsenicum* is not listed in the main rubric for perspiration, someone with a cold sweat may need that remedy if other symptoms also point to it. Similarly, many of the remedies listed under the subrubric "profuse" are not listed under the main one; but, once again, one of these remedies may be indicated if other symptoms point to it.
- It can also be seen that many of the remedies in "cold" are also in "profuse." If the person's perspiration has both characteristics, you would look at the remedies in both subrubrics:

Ant-t., Ars., Carb-v., China, Hep., Lyc., Merc., Sep., Verat. In order to choose between all these remedies you need another distinguishing characteristic of the ailment – for instance, vomiting, with diarrhea, which indicates *Ars., Nux v., Verat.* Of these, *Ars.* and *Verat.* are also indicated for cold and profuse perspiration (*Nux v.*

is hot). Now you have to choose between *Arsenicum* and *Veratrum album.* You then look at the Materia Medica, which gives the full description of both remedies. From this you should be able to decide which remedy is most similar to the ailment – the indicated homeopathic medicine.

BELOW *Use the Repertory Index and Materia Medica together to find the remedy best suited to your complaint.*

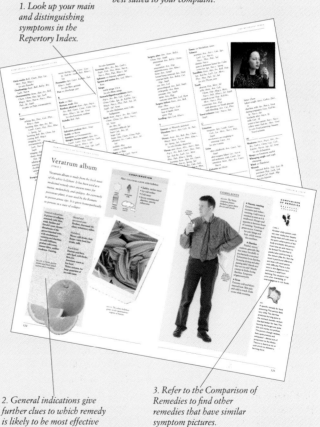

1. Look up your main and distinguishing symptoms in the Repertory Index.

2. General indications give further clues to which remedy is likely to be most effective

3. Refer to the Comparison of Remedies to find other remedies that have similar symptom pictures.

The Repertory Index

A

Abscesses: *Calc., Hep., Merc., Sil.*
Abdomen:
bloated: *Acon., Aloe, Arg-n., Ars., Bell., Bry., Calc., Carb-v., Cham., China, Lyc.*
flatulence: *Mag-p., Nat-m., Nux v., Sul.*
Abdominal cramps: *Aloe, Ars., Bry., Carb-v., Cham., Cocc., Coloc., Lyc., Mag-p., Nux v., Verat.*
better for:
bending back, arching: *Dios., Nux v.*
bending double: *Coloc., Mag-p., Podo.*
bending forward: *Coloc., Mag-p.*
pressure: *Coloc., Mag-p., Podo.*
Accidents:
injury: *Arn., Hyp.*
shock: *Acon., Arn.*
See also Wounds
Aching: *see* Pain, aching
Affectionate: *Phos., Puls.*
See also Emotions
Ailments from: *see* Causes, complaints from
Allergic reactions: *Apis, Rhus t., Urt-u.*
Angry: *Ars., Bell., Bry., Cham., Hep., Ign., Lyc., Nat-m., Nux v., Sep., Staph., Sul.*
See also Emotions
Anticipation: *Arg-n., Gels., Lyc.*
See also Emotions
Anxious: *Acon., Arg-n., Ars., Bell., Bry., Calc., Carb-v., Caust., China, Cocc., Lyc., Phos., Puls., Rhus t., Sep., Spong., Sul.*
during fever: *Acon., Ars., Ip., Sep.*
worse:
after midnight: *Ars.*
alone: *Ars., Phos.*
evening: *Calc., Carb-v., Sep., Sul.*
in bed: *Ars., Carb-v., Rhus t.*
waking: *Ars., Lach., Spong.*
See also Emotions

B

Babies:
collapse after long labor: *Carb-v.*
diaper rash: *Cal., Sul.*
teething: *Acon., Calc., Cham., Mag-p., Phyt., Sul.*
urine retention in newborn: *Acon.*
with diarrhea: *Calc., Cham., Podo., Sil., Sul.*
Back injuries: *see* Injuries
Bites and stings: *Apis, Hyp., Led., Rhus t., Urt-u.*
cold to touch: *Led.*
red, hot, swollen: *Apis*
shooting pains: *Hyp.*
Bladder problems: *see* Cystitis
Blood blisters: *Arn.*
Body temperature, general:
chilly: *Ant-t., Ars., Calc., Carb-v., Hep., Kali bic., Mag-p., Merc., Nux v., Phos., Sep., Sil., Verat.*
hot: *Apis, Arg-n., Puls., Sul.*
Boils: *Hep., Lach., Sil.*
Bones:
broken: *Arn., Ruta, Symph.*
pains in: *see* Injuries, bone
Breasts:
engorged: *Bell., Bry.*
hard, hot: *Bell., Bry.*
injuries: *Bell-p.*
inflammations, mastitis: *Bell., Bry., Hep., Merc., Phyt., Sil., Sul.*
nursing: *Phyt.*
painful: *Bell., Bry., Merc., Sil.*
red, streaked: *Bell.*
swollen: *Urt-u.*
Breastfeeding: *Bry., Calc., Cal., Cham., Phyt., Puls., Sep., Sil., Urt-u.*
excess milk: *Calc.*
exhaustion after: *Ars., Carb-v., China*
insufficient milk: *Calc., Puls., Urt-u.*
See also Nipples
Breath, offensive: *Ars., Hep., Merc., Puls., Sil.*
Bruises: *Arn., Ham., Ruta,*
external: *Arn., Ham.,*
internal: *Bell-p., Ruta*
Bronchitis: *Ant-t., Ars., Bry., Dros., Hep., Ip., Kali bic., Phos.*
See also Cough
Burns: *Cal., Canth., Caust., Urt-u.*
chemical: *Caust.*
minor: *Urt-u.*
second-degree: *Canth.*
third-degree: *Caust.*
Burning pains: *see* Pains, burning
Burping, belching: *Arg-n., Calc., Carb-v., Cham., China, Cocc., Ip., Lyc., Mag-p., Nat-m., Nux v., Phos., Puls.*

C

Causes, complaints from:
accidents: *Arn., Bell-p., Hyp.*
beer: *Aloe, Kali bic., Nux v.*
carbon monoxide poisoning: *Carb-v.*
coldness, chill: *Acon., Bry., Bell-p., Hep., Merc., Nux v., Phos., Rhus t., Sep., Spong.*
emotions:
anger: *Caust., Coloc., Ip., Staph.*
suppressed: *Staph.*
with indignation: *Staph.*
anticipation, anxiety: *Arg-n., Gels., Lyc.*
fright: *Acon., Ign.*
loss, grief: *Caust., Ign., Lach., Nat-m., Puls., Staph.*

love disappointment: *Ign., Lach., Nat-m., Staph.*

shock, bad news: *Gels.*

food poisoning: *Ars.*

injuries: *Arn., Hyp.*
  See also Injuries

loss of fluids: *Carb-v., China, Verat.*

sudden chill, when hot: *Bell-p.*

overexertion: *Arn., Mag-p., Rhus t., Ruta, Sul.*

overexposure: *Acon.*

overheated, becoming: *Acon., Bell., Bell-p., Bry., Lach., Nat-m., Puls.*

overindulgence, food/drink: *Ip., Nux v., Sul.*

sudden shock: *Acon.*

Cesarian, after: *Arn., Bell-p.,Cal., Hyp., Staph.*

Chest catarrh: *Ant-t.*

Chicken pox: *Apis, Merc., Puls., Rhus t., Sul.*

Childbirth: *Arn., Cal., Caul., Cham., Cimic., Gels., Hyp., Sep., Mag-m,. Puls., Ruta, Sep., Staph.*

after: *Arn., Hyp., Sep.*

blood loss during: *China*

exhaustion after: *Arn., China*

fear before: *Acon., Gels.*

intolerance to pain: *Cham., Cimic.*

labor pain:
  ceasing: *Arn., Cimic.*
  down thighs: *Caul., Cham.*
  exhausting: *Caul., Cimic.*
  false: *Caul., Gels.*
  fly across abdomen: *Caul., Cimic.*
  irregular: *Caul., Cham., Cimic., Puls.*
  weak: *Arn., Caul., Cimic., Puls.*
  prolapse after: *Ruta, Sep.*
  too fast: *Arn., Acon.*
  too slow: *Caul., Cimic., Gels., Puls.*
  See also Cesarian

Chilly: *see* Body temperature, chilly

Collapse: *Carb-v., Verat.*
in the elderly: *Carb-v.*

Colic: *Acon., Bry., Calc., Cham., China, Coloc., Dios., Ip., Lyc., Mag-p., Nux v., Staph., Sul.*

cramping pain: *Dios., Ip., Mag-p., Nux v., Staph., Coloc.*

in babies: *Cham., Coloc., Dios., Lyc.*

pain in waves: *Coloc.*

better:
  bending back, arching: *Dios., Nux v.*
  bending double: *Coloc., Mag-p.*
  hot drinks: *Nux v.*
  pressure: *Coloc.*
  warm bed: *Nux v.*
  warmth: *Mag-p.*

worse:
  after eating: *Nux v.*
  cold drinks, overheated: *Coloc.*

Common cold: *Acon., All-c., Ars., Bell., Bry., Calc., Carb-v., Euph., Gels.,*

eyes, nose, throat: *Hep., Kali bic., Lyc., Nat-m., Merc., Puls.*
  See also Ears

Conjunctivitis: *Apis, Bell., Euph., Puls.*
  See also Eye problems

Constipation: *Arg-n., Bry., Calc., Lyc., Nat-m., Sep., Sil., Nux v.*

Cough: *Acon., All-c., Ant-t., Bry., Calc., Carb-v., Caust., Euph., Hep., Ign., Ip., Kali bic., Phos., Puls., Sep., Spong., Sul.*

barking: *Acon., Bell., Bry., Dros., Hep., Spong.*

breathing, difficult: *Ant-t., Ars., Carb-v., Dros., Ip., Lyc., Nux v., Phos., Spong.*

chest, pain while coughing: *Arn., Bell., Bry., Caust., Dros., Gels., Ign., Kali bic., Phos., Spong.*

dry: *Acon., Ars., Bell., Bry., Calc., Caust., Cham., Dros., Gels., Hep., Ign., Ip., Lyc., Nux v., Phos., Puls., Spong., Sul.*

hoarse: *Acon., Caust., Ip., Spong.*

incessant: *Carb-v., Dros., Ip., Spong.*

loose: *Ars., Hep., Ip., Sep.*

must hold chest: *Arn., Bry., Dros.*

nausea with: *Ant-t., Ip., Puls.*

painful: *Acon., All-c., Bry., Caust., Hep., Lyc., Spong.*

phlegm:
  thick: *Carb-v., Hep., Kali bic., Sil.*
  profuse: *Ars., Calc., Carb-v., Euph., Hep., Kali bic., Lyc. Phos., Puls.*
  yellow: *Calc., Carb-v., Hep., Kali bic., Lyc., Phos., Puls., Sep.*

productive: *Carb-v., Euph., Hep., Kali bic., Lyc., Sep.*

rattling: *Ant-t., Caust., Hep., Ip., Lyc.*

suffocative: *Ant-t., Carb-v., Dros., Hep., Lach., Nux v., Sul.*

tickling: *Acon., All-c., Bell., Bry.,*

Calc., Caust., Cham., Dros., Ign., Ip., Kali bic., Lach., Lyc., Nat-m., Nux v., Phos., Puls., Rhus t., Spong.

unproductive: *Ant-t., Ars., Bry., Bell., Calc., Caust., Cham., Dros., Ign., Ip., Sep., Spong.*

vomiting, with: *Ant-t., Bry., Dros., Hep., Ip., Kali bic.*

whooping cough: *Ant-t., Arn., Bell., Carb-v., Dros., Ip.*
  See also Discharges

Croup: *Acon., Kali bic., Lach., Hep., Phos., Spong.*
  See also Cough

Cuts, grazes, lacerations: *Cal.*

Cystitis: *Acon., Apis, Ars., Canth., Caust., Lyc., Puls., Sep., Staph.*

urination, burning:
  after/end of: *Apis, Canth., Puls.*
  before: *Canth.*
  during: *Apis, Ars., Canth., Caust., Puls.*
  red sediment, with: *Canth., Lyc.*
  when not urinating: *Staph.*

D

Dental care:
after: *Arn., Cal., Hyp., Phos.,*
before: *Acon., Hyp.*

Diarrhea: *Acon., Aloe, Arg-n., Ars.,*

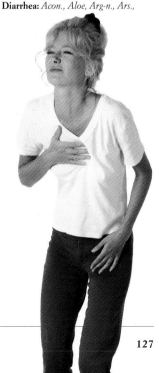

Calc., Carb-v., China, Coloc., Gels., Kali bic., Merc., Nux v., Podo., Puls., Sil., Staph., Sul., Verat.

after:

anger: *Coloc., Ip., Staph.*
beer: *Aloe, Kali bic.*
candy: *Arg-n.*
eating: *Ars., Ip., Nux v.*
stool: *Calc.*
burning: *Ars., Carb-v., Sul.*

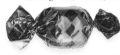

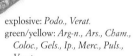

explosive: *Podo., Verat.*
green/yellow: *Arg-n., Ars., Cham., Coloc., Gels., Ip., Merc., Puls., Verat.*
involuntary: *Aloe, Verat.*
painful, severe: *Coloc., Verat.*
painless: *Aloe, Apis, China, Gels., Hep., Nat-m., Phos., Podo., Sil.*
teething with: *Calc., Cham., Podo., Sil., Sul.*
undigested food: *Ars., Calc., Cin., Sil.*
watery: *Arg-n., Ars., Calc., China, Nat-m., Phos., Puls., Rhus t., Sul., Verat.*

Discharges, general:

bland: *Puls.*
bloody: *Bry., Merc., Phos., Rhus t.*
burning: *Ars., Merc.*
clear: *Nat-m.*
excoriating, acrid: *Ars., Merc.*
like eggwhite: *Nat-m.*
green: *Kali bic., Puls., Merc.*
offensive: *Ars., Carb-v., Hep., Kali bic., Lyc., Merc., Sil., Sul.*
profuse: *China, Hep., Merc., Nat-m., Sil.*
pus: *Arg-n., Hep., Merc., Sil.*
sticky: *Kali bic., Lyc.*
thick: *Kali bic., Lyc., Merc., Puls.*
thin: *Ars., Merc., Nat-m., Sul.*
yellow: *Lyc., Kali bic., Merc., Puls., Sep., Sul.*

Dizziness, with nausea: *Cocc., Staph.*

Drinks:

aversion to: *Apis*
desires for:

alcoholic: *Acon., Arn., Lach., Led., Lyc., Nux v., Puls., Staph., Sep., Sul.*
beer: *Aloe, Arn., Bell., Caust., Cocc., Kali bic.*
coffee: *Nux v., Lach.*
cold: *Acon., Ant-t., Arg-n., Ars., Bell., Calc., Caust., Cham., China, Cocc., Mag-p., Merc., Phos., Rhus t., Sep., Verat.*
ice water: *Phos., Verat.*
lemon: *Bell.*
sour: *Arn., Ars., Cham.*
warm: *Ars., Hyp.*

Dryness, general: *Ars., Bell., Bry., Nat-m.*

Dry:

cough: *see* Cough
mucous membranes: *Bry., Spong.*
throat: *see* Throat, sore, dry

Dysentery/gastroenteritis: *Aloe, Ars., China, Coloc., Merc., Verat.*

E

Earache: *Acon., Apis, Bell., Calc., Cham., Hep., Kali bic., Lach., Lyc., Mag-p., Merc., Nux v., Puls., Sil., Sul.*

cause of complaint: *Arg-n., Caust., Cham., Cocc., Coloc., Gels., Ign., Lyc., Nat-m., Nux v., Sep., Staph.*
discharge, with: *Hep., Kali bic., Lyc., Merc., Puls., Sil.*
oversensitivity to noise: *Acon., Cham., Hep., Merc.*

Emotions:

affectionate: *Phos., Puls.*
alone, desires to be: *Ant-t., Bry., Gels., Ign., Nat-m., Rhus t.*
angry: *Ars., Bell., Bry., Cham., Coloc., Hep., Ign., Lyc., Nat-m., Nux v., Sep., Staph., Sul.*
anticipation: *Arg-n., Gels., Lyc.*
anxious: *Acon., Arg-n., Ars., Bell., Bry., Calc., Carb-v., Caust., China, Cocc., Ign., Lyc., Phos., Puls., Rhus t., Sep., Sil., Spong.*

carried, wants to be: *Cham., Puls.*
disappointed in love: *Ign., Nat-m., Staph.*
examination nerves: *Arg-n., Gels., Lyc.*
fearful: *Acon., Apis, Ars., Arg-n., Arn., Calc., Ign., Lyc., Phos., Puls., Sil., Spong.*

alone: *Apis, Arg-n., Ars., Lyc., Phos.*
dark: *Bell., Phos.*
death: *Acon., Apis, Ars., Calc., Cimic., Gels., Phos., Ruta*
flying, before: *Acon., Arg-n.*
touch: *Arn.*
home, wants to go: *Bry.*
indifferent, apathetic: *Carb-v., China, Gels., Nat-m., Phos., Sep., Verat.*
irritable: *Ant-t., Apis, Ars., Bry., Carb-v., Caust., Cham., Hep., Lyc., Mag-p, Nat-m., Nux v., Phos., Puls., Rhus t., Sil., Sep., Staph., Sul., Verat.*
quarrelsome: *Cham., Nux v., Sep.*
restless: *Acon., Apis, Arg-n., Ars., Bell., Caust., Cimic., Coloc., Dros., Lyc., Merc., Rhus t., Sil., Verat.*
sad: *Caust., Cimic., Ign., Nat-m., Rhus t.*
screaming: *Bell., Cham., Hep., Ip.*
sensitive: *Ars., Bell., Cham., Hep., Ign., Lyc., Nat-m., Nux v., Phos., Puls., Sil., Staph.*
sympathetic: *Caust., Phos., Puls.*
talks of pain: *Mag-p., Nux v.*
talkative: *Lach.*
tearful: *Apis, Calc., Carb-v., Caust.,*

Ign., Lyc., Nat-m., Puls., Rhus t.,
Ruta, Sep., Spong., Verat.
tearful, during fever: Acon., Bell.,
Puls., Spong.
Episiotomy: Hyp., Staph.
Exhaustion: Arn., Ars., Carb-v., China,
Gels., Mag-p., Phos., Sep., Verat.
from vomiting and diarrhea: Verat.
restlessness, with: Ars., Rhus t.
Eyes:
discharge:
bland: All-c., Bry.
burning: Caust., Euph., Merc.,
Sul.
profuse: All-c., Arg-n.
pus, with: Arg-n., Calc., Hep.,
Lyc., Merc., Puls.,
inflammation: All-c., Apis, Arg-n.,
Bell., Caust., Euph., Gels., Mag-
p., Merc., Puls., Rhus t., Ruta,
Sul.
problems after injury: Arn., Led.,
Ruta, Symph.
strain: Arg-n., Ruta

F

Face:
blue: Ant-t., Carb-v., Dros., Ip.,
Lach., Verat.
cold: Ant-t., Carb-v., Verat.
hot: Acon., Arn., Bell., Bry., Dros.
pale: Acon., Ant-t., Apis, Ars.,
Calc., Carb-v., Cham., China, Ip.,
Lyc., Verat.
puffy, swollen: Apis, Bry.
red: Acon., Apis, Bell., Bry., Cham.,
Gels., Lach., Phos., Rhus t., Sul.
Fanning, desires: Carb-v.
Fever: Acon., Ant-t., Apis, Ars., Bell.,
Bry., Cham., China, Dros., Gels.,
Hep., Ign., Ip., Lyc., Merc., Nat-m.,
Nux v., Phos., Puls., Rhus t., Sep., Sil.,
Sul., Verat.
(with) chill: Ars., Calc., Carb-v.,
China, Gels., Ip., Lach., Nux v.,
Puls., Verat.
(with) delirium: Bell.
dry: Acon., Apis, Bell., Bry., Nux v.,
Phos., Rhus t.
periodicity: Ars., China, Nat-m.
(with) sweat, profuse: Acon.,
Ant-t., Ars., Bry., Calc., China,
Hep., Merc., Phos.

(without) sweat: Ars., Bell., Bry.,
Gels.
(without) thirst: Bell., Gels., Phos.
Flatulence: Aloe, Arg-n., Carb-v.,
Cham., Chinà, Lyc., Mag-p.
after surgery: Carb-v., China
See also Abdomen, bloated
Food:
aversions:
beer: China, Nux v.
candy: Caust., Merc.
coffee: Bell., Cham., China, Ip.,
Nux v., Phos.
eggs: Sul.
fatty, rich food: Bry., Calc., Carb-
v., China, Hep., Ip., Merc., Nat-
m., Puls., Sep., Spong.
flatulent foods: Bry., China, Lyc.,
Coloc.
food, smell: Ars., Cocc., Ip., Sep.
fruit: China, Ip., Phos., Puls.
hot: China
meat: Arn., Bry., Calc., China,
Kali bic., Nux v., Puls., Sep.,
Sil., Sul.

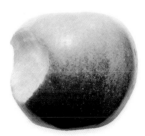

milk: Bry., Calc., China, Sep.,
Staph.
salty: Merc., Sep.
warm: Lach., Phos., Puls., Verat.
desires:
acids, food/drink: Acon., Ant-t.,
Bell., Bry., Kali bic., Verat.
bitter: Acon., Nat-m.
candy: Arg-n., Calc., China, Ip.,
Lyc., Rhus t., Phos., Sep.,
Staph., Sul.
chocolate: Phos., Sep.
eggs: Calc., Puls.
fatty: Nux v., Sul.
fruit: Verat.

ice cream: Calc., Phos.,
Puls.
lemons: Bell.
milk: Calc., Hyp., Rhus t.,
Sil.
onions: All-c., Bell-p.
salty: Arg-n., Carb-v., Caust.,
Nat-m., Phos., Verat.
sour/vinegar: Arn., Bell-p.,
Sep.
spicy: China, Phos., Sul.
See also Drinks, desires
poisoning: Ars., Carb-v., Urt-u.

G

German measles: see Rubella
Glands, swollen: Bell., Calc., Hep.,
Merc., Phyt., Rhus t., Sil.
See also Throat, Sore
Grief: see Emotions

H

Hallucinations:
during fever: Bell.
Hangovers: see Overindulgence
Hayfever: All-c., Ars., Euph., Kali bic.,
Nat-m., Nux v., Sul.
See also Nose, discharges; Eyes,
discharges; Common cold
symptoms
Head injuries: Arn., Hyp.
Headache: Acon., All-c., Arg-n., Arn.,
Bell., Bry., China, Gels., Hep., Ign.,
Ip., Kali bic., Lach., lyc., Nat-m., Nux
v., Phos., Puls., Mag-p., Merc., Rhus t.,
Sep., Sil., Sul.
better:
for holding head: Bry., Nat-m.,
Puls.
bursting: Acon., Bell., Bry., China,
Lach., Nux v., Puls., Sep.
eyestrain, from: Bry., Lyc., Nat-m.,
Nux v., Ruta, Sil.
(from) injury to the head: Arn.
nausea, with: Cocc., Ip., Nux v., Sul.
splitting: Bry., Nat-m.
(from) sun: Acon., Bell., Bry., Lach.,
Nat-m., Nux v.
throbbing: Acon., Ars., Bell.,
China, Ign., Lach., Lyc., Nat-m.,
Phos., Puls., Sep., Sil., Sul.
vomits after: Arg-n.

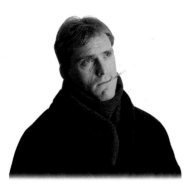

Headache: *(cont.)*
> coughing: *Bry., Lyc., Nat-m., Phos., Sul.*
> movement: *Bell., Bry., Hep., Nat-m., Sil.*
> See also Migraine

Hemorrhages: *Arn., Bell-p., China, Dros., Lach., Phos.*

Hemorrhoids: *Aloe, Ham., Hyp., Ign., Nux v., Sep.*
> external application: *Ham.*

Hives: *Apis, Ars., Rhus t., Urt-u.*

I

Indigestion: *Aloe, Arg-n., Ars., Calc., Carb-v., China, Ign., Lyc., Nat-m., Nux v., Puls., Sul.*

Influenza: *Acon., Ars., Bry., Gels., Ip., Nux v., Rhus t., Sul.*
> gastric: *Ars., Bry., Ip., Nux v.*

Injuries:
> bleeding freely: *Acon., Bell., Lach., Phos.*
> bones: *Arn., Calc., Ruta, Symph.,*
> bruising: *Arn., Bell-p., Ham., Ruta*
> external: *Arn., Cal., Hyp., Led., Ruta, Sil.*
> fingers, ends: *Hyp.*
> internal: *Arn., Bell-p., Staph.,*
> joints: *Arn., Bry., Calc., Rhus t., Ruta*
> nerves: *Arn., Hyp.*
> shock after: *Acon., Arn.*
> spine, fingers: *Hyp.*
> splinters, foreign bodies: *Hep., Hyp., Sil.*
> sports, exercise: *Arn., Bry., Led., Rhus t., Ruta, Symph.*
> wounds: *Arn., Cal., Led., Sil., Staph.*

Insect bites, stings: *see* Bites, Stings
Insomnia: *Ars., Cham., Ign., Lyc., Nux v., Rhus t.*
Irritable: *see* Emotions

J

Jetlag: *Arn.*
Joints:
> inflammations: *Apis, Bry., China, Led., Rhus t., Ruta*
> pains: *Arn., Apis, Bell-p., Bry., Calc., Caul., China, Kali bic., Lach., Led., Phyt., Rhus t., Ruta*
> swollen: *Apis, Bry., Lach., Led., Puls., Rhus t.*
> movement aggravates: *Bry., Led.*
> movement relieves: *Rhus t.*

Labor pains: *see* Childbirth
Laryngitis: *Acon., Arg-n., Bell., Calc., Caust., Hep., Kali bic., Phos., Puls., Spong.*
> See also Throat, sore

M

Mastitis: *see* Breasts
Measles: *Acon., Apis, Arn., Ars., Bell., Bry., Carb-v., Cham., China, Gels., Puls., Rhus t., Sul.*
Men, genitals: *Canth., Carb-v., Caust., Kali bic., Puls., Rhus t., Staph.*
> See also Prostatitis
Migraine: *Arg-n., Bell., Gels., Ign., Ip., Kali bic., Lach., Nat-m.*
> dim vision: *Gels., Lach.*
Modalities, better:
> air:
>> fresh (windows open): *Acon., Arg-n., Carb-v., Lach., Lyc., Puls., Rhus t., Sul.*
>> open (outside): *All-c., Aloe, Bry., Carb-v., Dros., Ip., Lach., Puls., Sul.*
> bathing: *Euph.* (eyes), *Puls.*
> breathing deeply: *Ign.*
> burping: *Carb-v., Lyc.*
> busy: *Sep.*
> carried: *Cham.*
> changing position: *Arn., Rhus t.*
> cold:
>> applications: *Apis, Bell-p., Led.*
>> bathing: *Arn., Led.*

> drinks: *All-c., Aloe, Caust., Ip., Lach., Phos., Phyt., Puls.*
> company: *Arg-n., Ars.*
> cool: *All-c., Aloe, Apis, Arg-n., Led., Phos.*
> crying: *Puls.*
> damp: *Caust.*
> discharges: *Lach., Nux v.*
> dry weather: *Bry., Calc., Caust., Phyt., Sul.*
> eating: *Phos., Sep.*
> exercise, vigorous: *Sep.*
> fanning: *Carb-v., Dros., Ip., Lach.*
> heat/warmth: *Ars., Calc., Canth., Caul., Caust., China, Hep., Ign., Kali bic., Mag-p., Nux v., Rhus t., Ruta, Sep., Sil., Staph.*
> hot applications: *Ars., Bry., Rhus t.*
> humid weather: *Hep., Nux v.*
> loose clothes: *Carb-v., China, Lach.*
> lying: *Arn., Cocc., Euph.*
>> quietly: *Hyp.*
>> still: *Bry., Led.*
> motion:
>> continued: *Rhus t.*
>> gentle: *Ars., Bell-p., Caust., Cimic., Kali bic., Lyc., Mag-p., Puls., Rhus t., Ruta, Sul.*
>> vigorous: *Sep.*
> pressure: *Bry., Coloc., Dros., Mag-p., Sep.*
>> hard: *China, Lach., Mag-p., Sil.*
> rest: *Acon., Bell., Bry., Canth., Led., Merc., Nat-m., Staph.*
> rubbing: *Canth., Urt-u.*
> sleep: *Phos.*
> swallow: *Ign., Lach.*
> sweating: *Gels., Nat-m., Rhus t.*
> urination: *Gels., Sil.*
> warm:
>> bed: *Ars., Caust., Hep., Lyc., Mag-p., Rhus t.*
>> drinks: *Hep., Lyc., Nux v., Rhus t., Spong., Verat.*

Modalities, worse:
> air, open (outside): *Caul., Cocc., Hep., Merc., Nux v., Sil., Sul.*
> alcohol: *Cham., Lach., Led., Nux v.*
> bathing: *Sul.*
> beginning movement: *Rhus t.*
> bending forward: *Bry.*
> candy: *Arg-n.*
> cold: *Ars., Bell-p., Caust., Cham., China, Cimic., Hyp., Mag-p.,*

Merc., Nux v., Phos., Puls.,
Rhus t., Ruta, Sep., Sil., Staph.
  bathing: Bell-p., Mag-p., Sil.,
  Urt-u.
  drinks: Ars., Bell-p., Canth.,
  Mag- p., Rhus t., Sil., Verat.
  damp: All-c., Calc., Cimic.,
  Gels., Kali bic., Mag-p.,
  Merc., Phyt., Rhus t., Sil.
  dry: Acon., Caust., Hep., Ip.,
  Mag-p., Spong.
coughing: Bry.
damp: Ant-t., Ars., Calc., Gels., Ip.,
  Merc., Rhus t.
drafts: Bell., Caust., China, Euph.,
  Rhus t., Sil., Sul.
eating/drinking: Aloe, Arg-n., Arn.,
  Ars., Cocc., Ip., Nat-m., Nux v.,
  Staph.
exertion: Ars., Calc., Carb-v., Cocc.,
  Nat-m., Staph., Sul.
fruit: China, Ip., Verat.
heat/warmth: Apis, Ars., Bry.,
  Carb-v., Cimic., Dros., Euph., Ip.,
  Lach., Led., Lyc. Merc., Nat-m.,
  Puls., Sul.
head wet, becoming: Bell.
hot weather: Acon., Aloe, Apis,
  Bell., Bry., Gels., Kali bic., Lach.,
  Nat-m., Podo., Puls.
loss of fluids: Carb-v., China, Verat.
lying down: Dros., Merc., Rhus t.,
  Ruta
milk: Calc., China, Mag-p., Sil.
movement: Bry., Caul., China,
  Cimic., Cocc., Gels., Hyp., Led.,
  Phyt., Spong.
  first movement: Rhus t., Ruta
noise: Bell., Cham., China, Sil.
pressure: Apis, Coloc., Hep., Hyp.,
  Lach., Lyc., Merc.
rest: Puls., Rhus t., Ruta, Sep.
sleep: Arn., Euph., Lach., Spong.
smell: Ip.
See also Nausea
sun: Bell., Gels., Nat-m.,
sweating: Gels., China, Merc.,
  Verat.
thunderstorms: Phos.
Time:
  midnight: Acon., Dros.
  1–2 a.m.: Ars.
  2–3 a.m.: Kali bic.
  4 a.m.: Caust., Nux v.

  early morning: Aloe, Sul.
  morning: Nat-m.
  11 a.m.: Sul.
  3 p.m.: Apis
  4–8 p.m.: Lyc.
  9 p.m.: Bry.
  evening: All-c., Puls.
  night: Hep., Led., Mag-p., Merc.,
    Phyt., Rhus t., Ruta, Sep., Sul.
tobacco: Ign., Nux v., Spong.
touch: Acon., Apis, Arn., Bell.,
  Bell-p., Bry., Canth., Cham.,
  China, Ham., Hyp., Ign., Lach.,
  Led., Mag-p., Nux v., Phos., Sep.,
  Sil., Staph.
uncovering: Hep., Mag-p., Nux v.,
  Rhus t., Sil.
warm:
  drinks: Phos.
  room: Ant-t., Apis, Arg-n., Bry.,
  Carb-v., Puls., Sul.
See also Causes, complaints from

Motion sickness: Cocc., Staph.
  See also Travel sickness
Mumps: Acon., Apis, Bell., Carb-v.,
  Lach., Lyc., Merc., Phyt., Puls.,
  Rhus t., Staph., Sul.
Muscular/skeletal: Apis, Bry., Calc.,
  Led., Lach., Mag-p., Phyt., Rhus t.,
  Ruta
  See also Injuries; Joints

N

Nausea: Ant-t., Cocc., Coloc., Ip., Nux
  v., Phos., Puls., Sep., Staph., Verat.
  (with) bleeding: Ip.
  eating, better for: Sep.
  (with) hunger: Ign.
  pregnancy: Cimic., Cocc., Kali bic.,
    Puls., Sep.
Nerves: Bell., Gels., Hyp., Mag-p.
Nervous: Arg-n., Ars., China, Cocc.,
  Ign., Rhus t.
  See also Emotions, anxious
Nettle stings: Urt-u.
Neuralgia: Acon., Bell., Caust., Cham.,
  Mag-p., Nux v.
Nightmares: Bell., Calc., Ign.
Nipples:
  cracked: Calc., Cal.
  inflamed: Cham.
  ulcerated: Sil.

Nose:
  blocked: All-c., Ars., Bry., Calc.,
  Carb-v., Gels., Hep., Ip., Kali bic.,
  Lyc., Merc., Nat-m., Nux v.,
  Phos., Puls., Sul.
  discharge from:
    bland: All-c., Puls.
    burning: All-c., Ars., Euph.,
    Gels., Lyc., Merc., Sul.
    green: Kali bic., Merc., Phos.
    offensive: Hep., Kali bic., Merc.
    profuse: All-c., Ars., Kali bic.,
    Merc., Nux v., Phos.
    stringy: Kali bic.
    thin, watery: All-c., Ars., Gels.,
    Nat-m., Sul.
    thick: Hep., Kali bic.
    white: Nat-m.
    yellow: Calc., Kali bic., Lyc.,
    Merc., Phos.
Nosebleed: Arn., Carb-v., Ham., Lach.,
  Phos.
  (with) whooping cough: Arn.,
    Dros., Ip., Phos., Puls., Sul.

O

Onset:
  gradual: Ant-t., Bry., Calc., Gels.,
  Kali bic., Lyc.
  sudden: Acon., Apis, Bell., Canth.,
  Coloc., Hep., Ip., Lach., Phyt.,
  Verat.

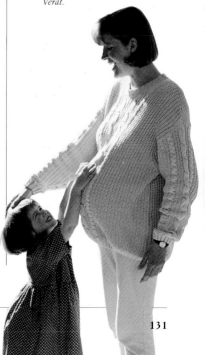

Otitis media: *Bell., Cham., Hep., Lyc., Merc., Puls., Rhus t.*
　See also Earache

Overheating: *Acon., Bell., Bell-p., Bry., Lach., Nat-m.*

Oversensitivity: *Acon., Apis, Ars., Bell., Cham., China, Hep., Ign., Lach. Mag-p., Merc., Nat-m., Nux v., Phos., Puls., Sil., Staph.*
　to pain: *see* Pain, oversensitivity

P

Pain:
　aching: *Bry., Dros., Gels., Phyt., Rhus t., Ruta*
　burning: *Aloe, Apis, Ars., Bry., Canth., Caust., Hyp., Phos., Rhus t., Spong., Sul.*
　bursting: *Bell., Bry., China, Sep.*
　cutting: *Bell., Mag-p.*
　dragging: *Sep.*
　oversensitivity to: *Cham., Ign., Lach., Nux v., Phos., Sep., Sil., Staph.*
　stinging: *Apis, Mag-p., Sil.*
　sharp, shooting: *Caul., Bell., China, Hep., Hyp., Led., Merc., Sep.*
　talking about: *Mag-p.*
　tearing: *Cham., Merc., Rhus t.*
　throbbing: *Bell., China, Sep.*
　violent, intense: *Acon., Bell., Hep., Cham., Mag-p., Merc., Nux v.*

Perspiration: *Calc., Merc., Sil., Verat.*
　absent during fever: *Ars., Bell., Bry., Gels.*
　cold: *Ant-t., Ars., Carb-v., China, Cocc., Hep., Ip., Lyc., Merc., Sep., Verat.*
　hot: *Acon., Cham., Ign., Ip., Nux v., Sep.*
　profuse: *Ant-t., Ars., Calc., Carb-v., China, Hep., Lyc., Merc., Phos., Sep., Sil., Sul., Verat.*

Pregnancy:
　hemorrhoids:
　　after: *Ham., Ign., Lach., Podo., Puls., Sep., Sul.*
　　during: *Ham., Lach., Nat-m., Nux v., Sep., Sul.*
　nausea: *see* Nausea:
　varicose veins during: *Bell-p., Ham., Puls.*
　vomiting: *see* Vomiting

worse during: *Caul., Cimic., Cocc., Ip., Kali bic., Lach., Puls., Rhus t., Sep.*

Prostatitis: *Apis, Caust., Kali bic., Puls., Rhus t., Staph.*
　See also Men, genitals

Pus: *see* Discharge, pus

R

Rash: *see* Skin

Rectum, weak: *Aloe*

Restless, physical: *Acon., Apis, Arg-n., Ars., Bell., Caust., Cimic., Coloc., Lyc., Merc., Rhus t., Sil., Sul., Verat.*
　See also Emotions, restless

Rubella: *Bell., Puls.*

S

Salivation, profuse: *Merc., Verat.*

Scalds: *see* Burns

Sensitive: *see* Oversensitivity

Shingles (herpes zoster): *Apis, Ars., Canth., Caust., Hep., Kali bic., Lach., Merc., Nat-m., Rhus t., Sul.*

Shock: *Acon., Arn., Hyp., Ign., Lach.*
　childbirth, after: *Acon.*
　surgery, after: *Acon.*

Side:
　right: *Apis, Bell., Canth., Caust., Hep., Lyc., Mag-p., Puls.*
　left: *Kali bic., Lach., Sep.*

Sinus problems:
　see Common cold
　see Headache
　see Nose, discharge

Skin: *Apis, Cal., Hep., Lach., Puls., Rhus t., Sil., Sul., Urt-u.,*
　bruises: *Arn., Ham., Ruta*
　cold: *Carb-v., Led., Verat.*
　hot: *Apis, Bell., Gels.*
　itchy: *Apis, Canth., Gels., Rhus t., Sul., Urt-u.*
　purple/blue: *Carb-v., Lach.*
　red: *Acon., Apis, Bell., Rhus t., Puls., Sul.*
　shiny: *Apis, Bell.*
　sunburn: *Cal., Urt-u.*
　　mild: *Cal.*
　　severe: *Urt-u.*
　See also Burns

Sleep, problems: *Acon., Calc., Ign., Rhus t.*

See also Insomnia

Sneezing: *All-c., Ars., Bry., Carb-v., Euph., Gels., Hep., Merc., Nat-m., Nux v., Phos., Puls., Rhus t., Sul.*

Splinters: *see* Injuries, splinters

Sprains and strains: *Bry., Led., Rhus t., Ruta*

Stings:
　nettle stings: *Urt-u.*
　See also Bites, stings

Stomach/digestive problems: *Acon., Arg-n., Ars., Bry., Calc., Carb-v., China, Coloc., Ign., Ip., Kali bic., Lyc., Mag-p., Nux v., Phos., Puls., Sep., Sil., Staph., Sul., Verat.*
　See also Abdomen, sore; Colic; Indigestion

Stool: *Acon., Arg-n., Ars., Bry., Caust., Cham., China, Lyc., Merc., Nux v., Sil., Verat.*
　dry: *Bry., Sil.*
　expulsion difficult: *Ign.*
　hard: *Calc., Bry., Sil.*
　large: *Calc.*
　loose: *Aloe, Cham., China, Podo.*
　offensive: *Ars., Carb-v., Merc., Sil., Sul.*
　sudden: *Aloe*
　watery: *see* Diarrhea

Sunburn: *see* Skin

Sunstroke: *Bell., Lach., Nat-m.*

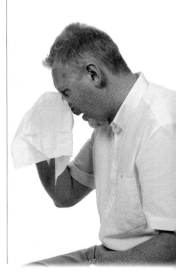

Surgery, after: *Arn., Acon., Bell-p., China, Hyp., Staph.*
  abdominal: *Arn., Bell-p., China, Staph.*
  amputation: *Arn., Hyp.*
  appendectomy: *Arn., Rhus t.*
  bone: *Arn., Symph.*
  breast/lump removal: *Arn., Ham.*
  cesarian birth: *Arn., Bell-p., Cal., Hyp., Staph.*
  eye: *Arn., Led.*
  gynecological: *Arn., Bell., Staph.*
  orthopedic: *Arn., Ruta*
  prostate: *Arn., Staph.*
  spine: *Arn., Hyp.*
  varicose veins: *Arn., Led., Ham.*
Surgery, before: *Acon., Arn., Bell., Hyp., Phos.*
  anxious: *Arg-n., Gels.*
  fear of death: *Acon.*
  spine: *Hyp.*
Swelling: *Apis, Led., Rhus t.*

T

Tetanus: *see* Wounds, puncture
Thirstless: *Ant-t., Apis, Gels., Ip., Puls., Verat.*
Thirsty: *Acon., Ars., Bell., Bry., Cham., Mag-p., Merc., Nat-m., Phos., Rhus t., Sil., Spong., Sul., Verat.*
  See also Drinks, desire for
Throat, sore: *Acon., All-c., Ant-t., Apis, Arg-n., Ars., Bell., Caust., Dros., Hep., Ign., Kali bic., Lach., Lyc., Merc., Phos., Puls., Rhus t., Spong.*
  burning: *Acon., Apis, Ars., Caust., Merc., Nat-m., Spong., Sul.*
  dry: *Acon., Bell., Bry., Calc., Gels., Kali bic., Lyc., Merc., Nat-m., Phos., Puls., Rhus t., Sil., Spong., Sul.*
  lump, sensation: *Gels., Ign., Lach., Lyc., Nat-m., Nux v., Phyt.*
  red: *Acon., Bell., Kali bic., Phyt.*
  swallowing, difficult:
    empty, painful: *Lach., Nux v.*
    pain better when: *Ign.*
    painful: *Ant-t., Apis, Bell., Hep., Lach., Merc., Phyt., Spong.*
  swollen: *Apis, Ars., Hep., Kali bic., Lach., Lyc., Merc., Phos., Puls., Phyt.*
  ulcerated: *Hep., Kali bic., Lyc., Merc., Phyt.*

Times: *see* Modalities, times
Tobacco
  aversion: *Arn., Ant-t., Calc., Ign., Lach., Lyc., Nat-m., Nux v., Phos., Puls., Sul.*
  desires: *Nux v.*
  pain in abdomen better for: *Coloc.*
  worse for: *Ign., Nux v., Spong.*
Tonsillitis: *Acon., Apis, Ars., Bell., Hep., Ign., Kali bic., Lach., Lyc., Merc., Phos., Phyt., Puls., Sil., Sul.*
  See also Throat, sore
Tooth:
  abscess: *Hep., Merc., Sil.*
  ache: *Acon., Arn., Calc., Cham., Hep., Mag-p., Merc., Nux v., Puls., Rhus t., Sil., Staph.*
  extends to ear: *Hep., Kali bic., Merc., Nux v., Phyt.*
  extraction: *Arn., Hyp.*
    with abscess: *see* Tooth abscess
    with bleeding: *Arn., Cal., Phos.*
Travel sickness: *Cocc., Nux v., Sep., Staph.*

U

Urination:
  frequent: *Apis, Canth., Caust., Gels., Lyc., Merc., Nux v., Puls., Staph.*
  involuntary on coughing or sneezing: *Caust., Sep.*
  See also Cystitis
Urine
  after childbirth: *Arn., Caust., Sep., Staph.*
  after surgery/labor: *Lyc., Nat-m.*
  red sediment, with: *Canth., Lyc.*
  retention: *Acon., Apis, Ars., Caust., Nat-m .*
Urticaria: see Hives

V

Varicose veins: *Bell-p., Ham.*
Voice, hoarse: *see* Laryngitis
Vomiting: *Acon., Ant-t., Ars., Bell., Bry., Calc., Cham., China, Coloc., Ign., Ip., Kali bic., Verat.*
  (after) anger: *Cham., Coloc., Ip., Nux v.*
  bile: *Ars., Cham., Ip., Nux v., Phos., Sep., Verat.*

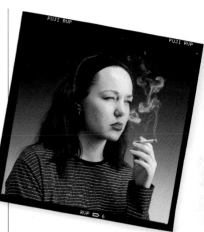

  bitter: *Cham.*
  (after) cough: *Ant-t., Carb-v., Dros., Ip.*
  diarrhea, with: *Ars., Nux v., Verat.*
  during pregnancy: *Cocc., Kali bic., Ip., Nux v., Sep.*
  headache after: *Arg-n., Ip.*
  milk: *Calc., Sil.*
  wants to but cannot: *Ant-t., Nux v.*
  yellow water: *Kali bic., Phos., Verat.*
  See also Food poisoning; Nausea; Travel sickness

W

Weakness: *Ant-t., Arg-n., Arn., Ars., Bry., Carb-v., China, Cocc., Gels., Kali bic., Nat-m., Sep., Sil., Verat.*
  See also Exhaustion
Weepy: *see* Emotions, tearful
Whooping cough: *see* Cough, whooping
Wind: *see* Flatulence
Wounds
  infected: *Bell-p., Hep., Led., Sil.*
  puncture: *Hyp., Lach., Led.*
  surgical: *Cal., Staph., Hyp.*
  See also Injuries

Home Medicine Chest

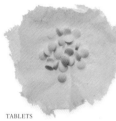

TABLETS

ABOVE, RIGHT, AND BELOW
*Homeopathic remedies come
in a number of forms.*

HOMEOPATHIC *remedies are excellent additions to any home
medicine chest, so that whatever situation arises you have
them on hand. All the remedies described in this book
are commonly used, though some are more specific for
certain ailments. A remedy such as* Arnica, *for example,
has such a broad range of use that you may want to have
more than one bottle in your home.*

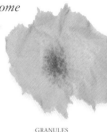

GRANULES

REMEDIES

Remedies in low potencies (6c, 30c) are readily available from many pharmacies and health food stores. Intermediate or higher potencies (6x, 12c, 200c, etc.) can be obtained from specialist homeopathic pharmacies that produce remedies for retail sale. Some pharmacies also sell prepared kits, such as the "First Aid Remedy Kit" produced by Helios or Ainsworths. Refer to Useful Addresses (*see pp. 140–1*).

AVAILABLE FORMS

Tablets

Tablets are sucked for about five minutes in the mouth, and then chewed.

There are also triturated tablets, that dissolve easily when placed under the tongue.

Granules

These are about the size of poppy seeds, and can easily be dissolved in a baby's mouth.

Powders

These are tipped under the tongue and allowed to dissolve.

All of the above are made by medicating lactose.

Sugar pillules

These have no dairy element, and they are therefore useful for those who are sensitive to dairy products.

Liquid

Liquid remedies are administered by dropper.

Creams, ointments, lotions

These are available for external use only. It is also possible to obtain remedies on a beeswax base, for those who are sensitive to lanolin.

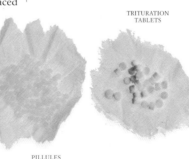

TRITURATION
TABLETS

PILLULES

WHERE TO OBTAIN YOUR REMEDIES

Natural and health food stores generally stock a wide range of remedies. Homeopathic pharmacies usually provide a set of remedies, or kit, specially assembled for home use, often at a discounted price.

HOW TO TAKE THE REMEDY

The medicines come in small bottles, which contain a number of sucrose tablets medicated with the tincture of the remedy, in the required potency. They are extremely easy to take; you simply allow the pill to dissolve slowly on or under the tongue. You should ideally take it with a "clean mouth," i.e. nothing else has been in the mouth for 15 to 20 minutes before taking the remedy, and leave another 15 to 20 minutes after taking it as well, so that no other substance interferes with its action. However, in cases of emergency, give the remedy regardless of this – it will probably work anyway. Always try to handle the remedy pill as little as possible.

MEDICINES FOR HOME USE

Here is a review of some of the remedies that may prove particularly valuable in your home medicine chest, listed according to general categories. In addition to the remedies that you take internally, you should include those that can be used topically.

Acute illnesses. These medicines are recommended for common colds, coughs, sore throats, indigestion, nausea, diarrhea, inflammations, childhood diseases, etc.
Aconite, Allium cepa, Aloe, Antimonium tartaricum, Apis, Argentum nitricum, Arnica, Arsenicum, Belladonna, Bryonia, Calcarea carbonica, Cantharis, Carbo vegetabilis, Causticum, Chamomilla, China, Colocynthis, Dioscorea, Drosera, Euphrasia, Gelsemium, Hamamelis, Hepar sulfuris calcareum, Ignatia, Ipecacuanha, Kali bichromium, Lachesis, Lycopodium, Magnesium phosphoricum, Mercurius, Natrum muriaticum, Nux vomica, Phosphorus, Phytolacca, Podophylum, Pulsatilla, Rhus toxicodendron, Sepia, Silica, Spongia, Staphisagria, Sulfur, Urtica urens, Veratrum album.

First aid. This group of medicines is particularly useful for minor accidents and injuries such as bruises, blows, falls, sprains, strains, cuts, wounds, fractures, etc. Anyone can benefit from these, especially children and those frequently engaged in sports and exercise.
Aconite, Apis, Arnica, internal

RIGHT *Touch the remedy pill as little as possible. To take a remedy, carefully tip the pill into the cap of the bottle.*

remedy and cream (on bruises, not open wounds), *Calendula,* cream, tincture, gel, ointment*, Cantharis, Carbo vegetabilis, Causticum, Hamamelis* internal remedy and cream or tincture, *Hypericum, Ledum, Rhus toxicodendron, Ruta, Staphisagria, Symphytum, Urtica urens* internal remedy and cream or tincture.

Also available are creams with mixtures, suitable for topical application, such as *Hypericum* and *Calendula,* and *Urtica* and *Calendula.*

Birth remedies: These remedies are invaluable aids during childbirth, and after. You will see that some of these remedies are in the other groups as well, because they have a wide spectrum of application.
Aconite, Arnica, Belladonna, Calendula, Caulophyllum, Cimicifuga, Gelsemium, Ignatia, Hypericum, Pulsatilla, Rhus toxicodendron, Sepia, Staphysagria.

Travel kit: Medicines to take with you when you travel. Here is a basic list, but you can always add to it if you feel you are prone to certain ailments requiring other remedies.

Aconite (acute fear, fear of flying, any sudden shock, the first sign of a cold, diarrhea from overheating), *Aloe* (traveler's diarrhea, if symptoms fit), *Apis* (insect bites), *Arnica* (any trauma, and exhaustion of jet lag; never leave home without it), *Arsenicum* (a specific remedy for food poisoning), *Belladonna* (ailments from sunstroke, such as headaches), *Calendula* (skin wounds, sunburn), *Carbo vegetabilis* (sudden collapse from inhalation of exhaust fumes), *Cocculus* (travel sickness), *Gelsemium* (fear of flying, if the symptoms fit), *Hypericum* (first aid remedy for injury to nerves), *Ledum* (insect bites, puncture wounds, especially if in danger of contracting tetanus), *Nux vomica* (overindulgence in food and drink; hangover), *Podophyllum* (diarrhea, if symptoms fit), *Rhus toxicodendron* (sprains, strains, urticaria), *Symphytum* (bone fractures, eye injuries), *Urtica urens* (urticaria).

Potencies: Ideally, have the remedies in both the 6c and 30c potencies. The one you use depends on the severity of symptoms (refer to section on dosage). The 6c potency is the most widely available in health stores and certain pharmacies. However, the 30c is a highly effective low potency to be recommended if you prefer to have only one potency.

CAUTION
Store your remedies in bottles, away from direct sunlight and any strong odors.

135

Sample Case Study

THIS CASE STUDY *shows how to use homeopathy in a first aid or acute situation. Look for the most important, identifying characteristics at that time. Listen to the symptoms that the patient describes. Where is the pain? What type? Does anything make it better or worse? Pressure? Heat? Cold? Closely observe the*

LEFT *Your daughter is normally a calm and happy child, with no fears.*

state of the patient, especially in children. Degrees of restlessness? Color of the face? General mood? Are pupils dilated? Then take the clearest, strongest symptoms to repertorize.

Your daughter wakes in the early hours of the morning, crying loudly and clearly in a great deal of pain.

When she was put to bed the previous night she was perfectly fine and happy. You notice her face is very red, and her whole body is very hot, so that you feel the heat radiating from her. Clearly she has a high fever, but she is not sweaty.

She puts her hand to her right ear, indicating that is where the pain is. She is very agitated, kicks the covers off, refuses your comfort, and pushes you away, does not wish to drink when offered.

She screams, through her tears, something about spiders being all over her bed and she is fearful of this. Normally she is a cheerful, independent, sweet, and mild-tempered child.

It is most likely your daughter has an ear infection. What are her symptoms?

- She was perfectly well the night before, and now has a high fever.
- She is very hot, and her face is red, but she is not sweaty.
- She is in a great deal of pain, from her infected ear; earache.
- She is in a terrible mood.
- She does not want to drink anything.
- She seems to imagine that she sees spiders on the bed.

RIGHT *She keeps tugging at her ear, indicating the source of her pain.*

BELOW LEFT *She is fearful of spiders crawling all over her bed.*

How do these symptoms translate to the language of the repertory?

- Onset, sudden
- Fever, dry and face, red (two symptoms)
- Earache
- Emotions angry, or restless
- Thirstless
- Hallucinations during fever

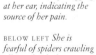

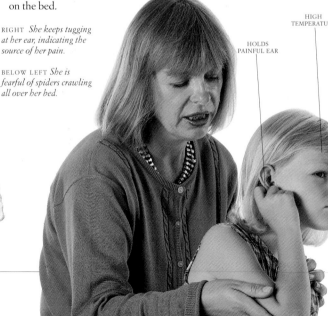

HIGH TEMPERATURE

HOLDS PAINFUL EAR

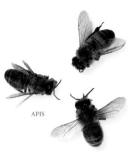

APIS

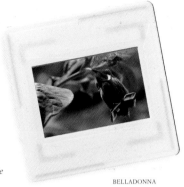

BELLADONNA

ABOVE AND RIGHT *Apis or Belladonna might be an appropriate remedy to try for symptoms such as those described here.*

Here you have seven clear and strong symptoms. If you look them up in the Repertory Index you find these remedies:

1 Onset sudden: *Acon., Apis, Bell., Canth., Coloc., Hep., Ip., Lach., Phyt., Verat.*

2 Fever dry: *Acon., Apis, Bell., Bry., Nux v., Phos., Rhus t.* (The symptom "Fever" has many remedies in it, and will not help you as much as the more precise symptom "Fever, dry.")

3 Face, red: *Acon., Apis, Bell., Bry., Cham., Gels., Lach., Phos., Rhus t., Sul.*

4 Earache: *Acon., Apis, Bell., Calc., Cham., Hep., Kali bic., Lach., Lyc., Mag-p., Merc., Nux v., Puls., Sil., Sul.*

5 Emotions angry: *Ars., Bell., Bry., Cham., Coloc., Hep., Ign., Lyc., Nat-m., Nux v., Sep., Staph., Sul.*

6 Thirstless: *Ant-t., Apis., Gels., Ip., Puls., Verat..*

7 Hallucinations during fever: *Bell.*

Belladonna would seem to be the best remedy as it is indicated in 6 out of 7 symptoms and is the only one for 7.

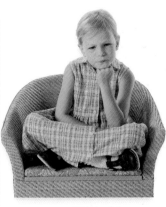

ABOVE *Your daughter wishes to be left alone and refuses a comforting hand.*

You then read the full description of *Belladonna* in the Materia Medica, which confirms your choice. The remedy picture fits the picture of the illness in many important respects.

You also see that *Belladonna* is thirsty, except during a fever.

If you had used just the first three symptoms, the remedies indicated would be:

Acon., Apis, and Bell. If your daughter was not hallucinating (mild as it was, you may not have noticed), how would you have chosen among these three particular remedies?

In reading the description of *Aconite*, you find that the emotional state is more fearful, less angry or restless. *Aconite* would be more thirsty, with a burning thirst.

Apis would appear to be very similar to *Belladonna*, with a right-sided earache, sudden onset, redness, and inflammatory state with dry heat, thirstless (aversion to water), restless, and irritable. You decide to give *Apis* 30c, one dose every half hour, because the progress of the illness is very rapid and the pain is intense, but after three doses she is not better. You decide then to give *Belladonna* 30c. After 15 minutes she is quieter, and seems drowsy. This is a good reaction, so you do not give any more doses. She falls asleep at last, and so do you! The next morning she is slightly worse again, so you repeat a dose of *Belladonna*. The fever is down, but she is still unwell. You continue to repeat the remedy only when you observe that she is not continuing to get better, that her rate of recovery has slowed down.

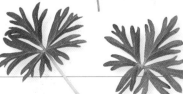

LEFT Aconite *would be given in cases similar to this, but when the mood is more fearful than angry.*

Glossary

A

Abdomen: the part of the body between the chest and the pelvis.

Abortion: spontaneous or abrupt termination of a pregnancy before full term.

Abscess: localized collection of pus caused by micro-organisms, usually with redness, heat, swelling, and pain.

Acrid: irritating, excoriating, bitter.

Acute: of sudden onset and brief duration.

Aggravation: symptoms become worse.

Appendicitis: inflammation of the appendix.

Aversion: intense dislike, usually referring to food and drink.

B

Boil: acute inflammation around a hair follicle.

C

Cesarian birth: delivery of the fetus by abdominal incision.

Catarrh: chronic inflammation of mucous membranes, with constant flow of thick mucus.

Chicken pox: acute infectious disease caused by a virus, with malaise, fever, and characteristic rash consisting of red elevated vesicles or blisters that crust over and come in crops.

Chronic: persisting for a long time; a state showing little or no change.

Coccyx: the last bone of the spine; the "tailbone."

Colic: acute but intermittent abdominal pain that gradually increases then decreases.

Concussion: condition resulting from a violent shock or blow.

Conjunctivitis: inflammation of the conjunctiva, the inner lining of the eyelids; "pink eye."

Constipation: abnormally infrequent or difficult bowel movements.

Constitutional: treatment based on the totality of a person's symptoms, including medical history, genetic makeup, physical, emotional, and mental symptoms.

Cramp: painful spasmodic muscular contraction.

Croup: inflammatory condition of larynx and trachea, usually of children, with laryngeal spasm, breathlessness, and difficult, noisy breathing.

Curettage: the scraping of tissue from a cavity, such as the uterus.

Cystitis: inflammation of the bladder.

D

Desires: intense preference, usually referring to food and drink.

Diarrhea: frequent evacuation of loose, watery stools.

Discharge: an excretion or substance evacuated from the body.

Dislocation: injury to joint, so that the ends of the opposed bone are no longer in connection with each other.

Distention: abnormal swelling.

Dosage: frequency of administration of the remedy.

E

Epidural: injection of local anesthetic into the epidural space, the region through which spinal nerves leave the spinal cord, for pain relief during childbirth or surgical operations.

Episiotomy: cut made in the vulva during childbirth, supposed to prevent tearing.

F

Fever: elevation of body temperature above normal.

Fibrous tissue: common connective tissue of the body.

Flatulence: gas or air in stomach or intestines; wind coming up or going down.

G

Gastric: pertaining to the stomach.

Gastroenteritis: inflammation of the mucous membranes of the stomach and the small intestines due to dietary error of presence of microbes.

Genital: pertaining to the organs of reproduction.

German measles: acute, infectious, eruptive fever, with pink rash and enlarged cervical glands; usually without complications, unless contracted during early months of pregnancy, when it may produce fetal deformities.

Glands: organ or structure capable of secretion, such as salivary or mammary; the lymph glands do not secrete but are concerned with filtration of lymph.

H

Hemorrhage: escape of blood from a ruptured blood vessel.

Hemorrhoid: varicose veins around the anus.

Hives: an allergic skin reaction characterized by many smooth, raised, pinkish, itchy weals which come up suddenly; nettlerash, urticaria.

Hyperactivity: excessive activity and distractibility.

Hypochondriacal: having excessive anxiety about one's health.

I

Incision: the result of cutting into the body with a sharp instrument.

Indigestion: a feeling discomfort in the stomach or abdomen.

Inflammation: protective tissue response to injury, infection, or irritation, characterized by heat, redness, swelling, and usually pain.

Insomnia: sleeplessness; inability to fall asleep.

L

Laceration: the result of tearing of tissues by blunt instrument.
Lactose: milk sugar.
Laryngitis: inflammation of the larynx.
Larynx: the organ of voice, located at the top of the trachea.

M

Macerated: finely chopped.
Mammary: pertaining to the breast.
Mastitis: inflammation of the breast.
Materia medica: information regarding the origins and properties of medicines.
Measles: acute, infectious viral disease characterized by fever, rash, and inflammation of the mucous membranes.
Menopause: the end of the period of possible sexual reproduction with cessation of menstrual periods.
Metastasis: the spread of disease from one part of the body to another.
Modality: factor which makes symptoms better or worse.
Mumps: acute infection of parotid salivary gland causing swelling of face and neck, occasionally other organs.

N

Nausea: feeling of sickness.
Neuralgia: affection of nerves, causing intense pain.

O

Orchitis: inflammation of a testis.
Otitis media: inflammation of the middle ear.

P

Paralysis: loss of nervous function to a part of the body.
Periosteum: the membrane which covers a bone.
Peritonitis: inflammation of the peritoneum, the membrane which lines the abdominal and pelvic cavities.
Pertussis: *see* **Whooping cough.**
Pharynx: the cavity at the back of the mouth.

Phlegm: the secretion of mucous expectoration from the lungs.
Photophobia: inability to expose the eyes to light.
Potency: the strength of the homeopathic remedy; the degree to which the homeopathic remedy has been diluted and succussed.
Prostatitis: inflammation of the prostate gland.
Proving: the process of testing a medicinal substance on healthy people in order to discover the symptoms it can elicit.
Pruritis vulva: the condition of itching of the vulva, the external female genitalia.
Puncture wound: a penetrating wound made by a sharp, pointed instrument.
Pus: a liquid formed in certain infections containing bacteria and white blood cells.

R

Remedy: the term commonly used in homeopathy to denote the homeopathic medicine.
Repertory: indexed arrangement of symptoms and the remedies which are know to produce or cure those symptoms.
Respiratory: pertaining to breathing; the respiratory system comprises the nose, pharynx, larynx, trachea, bronchi, and lungs.
Rheumatism: disorder of the connective tissue, usually with pain, stiffness, and swelling of muscles and joints.
Rubella: *see* **German measles.**

S

Sciatica: pain in the sciatic nerve, extending from buttock to back of thigh, calf, and foot.
Septic: putrefying due to presence of disease, producing bacteria.
Shingles: an acute disease caused by the chicken pox virus and characterized by severe pain and extremely sensitive vesicles on an area of skin limited by its nerve supply.

Shock: sudden and disturbing mental or physical impressions; also a state of collapse characterized by pale, cold, sweaty skin, rapid, weak pulse, faintness, dizziness, and nausea.
Sinusitis: inflammation of the sinuses.
Spasm: sudden, violent involuntary muscular contractions.
Sprain: injury to the soft tissue surrounding a joint, resulting in discoloration, swelling, and pain.
Sputum: spittle.
Strain: damage due to excessive muscular effort.
Succussion: vigorous shaking of the remedy mixture as part of the preparation of a homeopathic remedy.
Susceptibility: the aspect of the individual which succumbs to disease-causing influences.
Symptom: perceived changes in sensations and functions of body or mind, indicating disease or injury.

T

Thrush: fungal infection of throat or vagina.
Trachea: windpipe.
Trauma: physical injury or wound; disturbing experience which causes emotional or psychological upset.
Trituration: easily dissolvable.

U

Ulcer: open sore on internal or external surface of the body.
Urticaria: pale or red elevated patches with severe itching; nettle rash; hives.
Uvula: soft, cone-shaped, fleshy mass hanging centrally from soft palate at back of the mouth.

V

Varicose veins: dilated veins; valves become weak, so blood flow is reversed.

W

Whooping cough: infectious disease characterized by coryza, bronchitis, and violent spasmodic cough; attacks of violent coughing that end in an inspiratory whoop; pertussis.

Further Reading

BLACKIE, Dr. Margery,
The Challenge of Homeopathy
(Unwin Paperbacks, 1981)

BLACKIE, Dr. Margery,
Classic Homeopathy
(Beaconsfield Publishers, 1990)

BODMAN, Dr. Frank,
*Clinical Homeopathy:
Insights into Homeopathy*
(Beaconsfield Publishers, 1990)

BORLAND, Dr. Douglas,
Homeopathy in Practice
(Beaconsfield Publishers, 1982)

CASTRO, Miranda,
*Miranda Castro's Homeopathic Guides:
Homeopathy for Mother and Baby*
(Pan, 1996)

CASTRO, Miranda,
*Miranda Castro's Homeopathic Guides:
The Complete Homeopathic Handbook*
(Pan, 1996)

CHAITOW, Leon,
*Vaccination and Immunisation,
Dangers, Delusions and Alternatives*
(C. W. Daniel, 1987)

COULTER, Harris,
*Homeopathic Science
and Modern Medicine*
(North Atlantic Books, 1981)

CUMMINGS, Stephen,
and ULLMAN, Dana,
*Everybody's Guide to
Homeopathic Medicines*
(Victor Gollancz, 1990)

CURTIS, Susan,
*Handbook of Homeopathic
Alternatives to Immunisation*
(Winterpress, 1994)

GARION-HUTCHINGS,
Nigel and Susan,
*The New Concise
Guide to Homeopathy*
(Element Books, 1993)

GEMMELL, Dr. David,
Everyday Homeopathy
(Beaconsfield Publishers, 1987)

GIBSON, Dr. D. M.,
*First Aid Homeopathy
in Accidents and Ailments*
(British Homeopathic Association,
1988)

HAYFIELD, Robin,
Homeopathy for Common Ailments
(Gaia Books, 1991)

HERSCU, Paul,
*The Homeopathic
Treatment of Children*
(North Atlantic Books, 1991)

KOEHLER, Gerhard,
*The Handbook of Homeopathy:
Its Principles and Practice*
(Thorsons Publishers, 1986)

LESSELL, Dr. Colin B.,
*World Traveller's
Manual of Homeopathy*
(Saffron Walden, 1993)

McTAGGART, Lyn,
The Vaccination Bible
(Brian Hubbard, 1997)

MOSCOWITZ, Richard, M.D.,
*Homeopathic Medicines
for Pregnancy and Childbirth*
(North Atlantic Books, 1992)

NEUSTAEDTER, Randell,
*The Vaccine Guide:
Making an Informed Choice*
(North Atlantic, 1996)

PANOS, Maesimund, and HEIMLICH,J.,
Homeopathic Medicine at Home
(Corgi, 1980)

PRATT, Dr. Noel,
Homeopathic Prescribing
(Beaconsfield Publishers, 1985)

SANKARAN, Rajan,
The Spirit of Homeopathy
(Sankaran Rajan Publishers,
Bombay, 1981)

SHEPHERD, Dr. Dorothy,
Homeopathy for the First Aider
(C. W. Daniel, 1953)

SHEPHERD, Dorothy,
Homeopathy in Epidemic Diseases
(Health Science Press, 1967)

SHEPHERD, Dorothy,
The Magic of the Minimum Dose
(Health Science Press, 1967)

SHEPHERD, Dorothy,
More Magic of the Minimum Dose
(Health Science Press, 1967)

SMITH, Trevor,
*Homeopathic Medicine:
A Doctor's Guide to Remedies
for Common Ailments*
(Thorsons Publishers, 1986)

SPEIGHT, Phyllis,
Homeopathy for Emergencies
(Health Science Press, 1984)

SPEIGHT, Phyllis,
Homeopathic Treatment for Children
(Health Science Press, 1993)

ULLMAN, Dana, M.P.H.,
The Consumer's Guide to Homeopathy
(G. P. Putnam's Sons, 1995)

VITHOULKAS, George,
Homeopathy: Medicine of the New Man
(Arco Publishing Inc., 1983)

VITHOULKAS, George,
The Science of Homeopathy
(Thorsons Publishers, 1993)

WELLS, Henrietta,
Homeopathy for Children
(Element Books, 1993)

WRIGHT HUBBARD, Dr. Elizabeth,
Homeopathy as an Art and Science
(Beaconsfield Publishers, 1990)

Supplier of Homeopathic Books:
Minerva Books,
173 Fulham Palace Road,
London W6 8QT
(most comprehensive supplier)

Useful Addresses

U.S.A

North American Society of Homeopaths
1122 East Pike Street,
#1122
Seattle
WA 98122
Tel: 206 720 7000
Fax: 206 329 5684
email: nashinfo@aol.com

Hahnemann Homeopathic Pharmacy
828 San Pablo Avenue
Albany
California CA 94706
Tel: 510 527 3003
Fax: 510 524 2447

U.K.

Society of Homeopaths
4a Artizan Road
Northampton NN1 4HU
Tel: 01604 621400
Fax: 01604 622622
email: info@homeopathy-soh.org
Send S.A.E. for full list of Registered Homeopaths

Helios Homeopathic Pharmacy
97 Camden Road
Tunbridge Wells
Kent TN1 2QR
Tel: 01892 537254
Fax: 01892 546850
Email: helios@pharmacy.co.uk
International mail order services available, and homeopathic kits including remedies discussed in this book.

Ainsworth's Homeopathic Pharmacy
38 New Cavendish Street
London W1G 8TS
Tel: 020 7935 5330
Mail order service available.

AUSTRALIA/NEW ZEALAND

The Australian Association of Professional Homeopaths
80 Essenden Road
Anstead
Queensland 4070
Tel/Fax: 61 732026517

Australian Homeopathic Association
6 Cavan Avenue
Renown Park
SA 5008
Tel/Fax: 61 8 8346 3691
Email: smick@smartchat.net.au

New Zealand Council of Homeopaths
PO Box 51-195
Tawa
Wellington
New Zealand
Tel: 64 025 640 0792

New Zealand Homeopathic Society
P.O. Box 67-095
Mount Eden
Auckland
New Zealand
Tel: 09 630 5458

Similimum Pharmacy
P. O. Box 10889
290 Panama Street
Wellington
New Zealand
Tel: 04 499 9242
Fax: 04 499 5245
Email: orders@arnica.co.nz

Index